JAUNDICE DURING PREGNANCY

WITH SPECIAL EMPHASIS ON

RECURRENT JAUNDICE DURING PREGNANCY

AND ITS DIFFERENTIAL DIAGNOSIS

BY

URS PETER HAEMMERLI

Springer Science+Business Media, LLC

ALSO PUBLISHED AS SUPPLEMENT NO. 444 TO ACTA MEDICA SCANDINAVICA 1966.

ISBN 978-0-387-90001-8   ISBN 978-1-4757-5621-0 (eBook)
DOI 10.1007/978-1-4757-5621-0
Library of Congress Catalog Card Number 67-21050

Title No. 1430

INDEX

FOREWORD

During the years 1959 to 1964 we had the occasion to observe personally 5 patients with recurrent intrahepatic cholestasis of pregnancy and to follow them through multiple gestations. These cases, together with a sixth case discovered in the hospital files, have been described in detail elsewhere (Haemmerli and Wyss). The perusal of the literature during the preparation of that manuscript soon revealed, that not all cases of recurrent jaundice *during* pregnancy could be due to recurrent jaundice *of* pregnancy i.e. the cholestatic form. It also became apparent that an attempt at a differential diagnosis of recurrent jaundice during pregnancy has never been made and that many conflicting statements in the literature on recurrent jaundice during pregnancy originate in the lack of clear definitions.

The present paper attempts to fill this need. In order to achieve our purpose it has become necessary to present in a first part a brief review of the changes in so-called liver function tests during uncomplicated pregnancy and in a second part a general review of jaundice during pregnancy. The third and main part will be devoted to a description and definition of recurrent intrahepatic cholestasis *of* pregnancy on the basis of all verified cases in the world literature including our own patients and to a description of all other disorders which may present as recurrent jaundice *during* pregnancy. We believe that the literature in the third part is as complete as it possibly can be. The first two parts had to be somewhat restricted in content, and while they—as we hope—will present a fair summary of the present state of knowledge, not all papers covering the respective topics could be included.

Our interest in jaundice during pregnancy has been stimulated during our work as medical consultant and gastro-enterologist to the Department of Obstetrics, Zürich University Hospital, and I wish to gratefully acknowledge the continuing help and encouragement received from its chief, Professor E. R. Held, his co-worker Dr. H. I. Wyss, and from my chief, Professor P. H. Rossier, head of the Department of Medicine, Zürich University Hospital.

I. The liver in normal pregnancy

The liver performs its function well during gestation. Tests and laboratory determinations usually employed to evaluate liver function and liver disease deviate, however, not infrequently from the normal in healthy pregnant women. These disturbances are rarely severe, surpassing the accepted upper limit of normal for non-pregnant females only slightly. They are on the main more common in the later weeks of gestation and are usually rectified after delivery.

The knowledge of the "physiological" derangements is important for any physician evaluating a women with jaundice during pregnancy. In the non-pregnant state there exists for every test an accepted division line between a normal and a pathological result. It is probably wise to follow Friedberg's suggestion to form a third intermediary group of test results in pregnant women: those lying above the upper limit of normal for non-pregnant subjects, but lying below the highest observed values in uncomplicated pregnancies. As only a certain percentage of pregnant females surpass the non-pregnant norm, this intermediary group may then be truely "normal", or may have a pathological significance.

Reviews of liver function in uncomplicated pregnancy have been attempted by Holmer 1927, Vignes 1935, Dietel 1936, Williams 1952, Dieckmann 1952, Lichtman 1953, Thorling 1955, Hoynck Van Papendrecht 1957, Richman 1960 and Friedberg 1960, 1962, 1963. A fair summing-up has been made by Cross in 1929: "The liver is the largest, the most abused, the most neglected, one of the most important, and the least understood organ of the body".

Liver palpation

Palpation of the liver can be difficult in the later weeks of gestation, when the liver may be forced upwards, backwards and to the right by the enlarged uterus. A normal liver is rarely palpable towards term. When it is felt, liver disease or congestive heart failure should be suspected.

Spider angiomas and palmar erythema

Bean et al. carefully examined all women in a prenatal clinic during one year. They found spider angiomas in 66.6 % of 484 white and in 11.4 % of 759 negro pregnant females. The control incidence was 12 % among 58 non-pregnant white females with children and 14.9 % among 295 white soldiers. In the same pregnancy groups 62.5 % of white and 35 % of negro females had palmar erythema. There was an overlap in the occurrence of spider angiomas and palmar erythema in about two thirds of each group. Spider angiomas occurred as early as the second month of gestation with a sharp incidence rise between the 2nd and 5th month and but a slow rise thereafter. During pregnancy the single spider angioma may increase in size and new ones may appear in the second and third trimester. Most disappear after delivery.

Bean et al.'s study is the result of a meticulous search for these skin changes. It is not surprising that they are usually not noted by the more hasty observer and that they are rarely mentioned in obstetric textbooks.

Histological changes in liver biopsies

In 1907 Hofbauer described as typical histological changes of the liver during pregnancy: centrolobular fatty degeneration, decreased glycogen content, centrolobular bile stasis and ectasia of the centrolobular veins and capillaries. He coined the term "Schwangerschaftsleber". His opinion was based on 4 postmortem examinations of pregnant women dying at term: three from pulmonary emboli and one from exsanguination during delivery. This concept was challenged in 1910 by Schickele but still kept appearing in the literature up to 1945. It is now clear that Hofbauer's observations were due to unrelated and terminal pathology in his 4 cases.

In 1945 Ingerslev and Teilum performed liver biopsies in 17 females during delivery. They found some variation in the size of liver cells and nuclei, occasionally small lymphocytic infiltrations in the portal spaces, and sometimes a mild vacuolar accumulation of fat in the centrolobular area which was more pronounced than in their 6 nonpregnant controls. Otherwise the liver histology

was considered normal. In 1947 Nixon et al. biopsied 9 pregnant females and found only minor nonspecific histological changes. These consisted in an occasional variation in the shape of liver cells, in an increase in the number of large nuclei, in some irregularities of the nuclei, and in an increased glycogen content of the cytoplasm. In the same year Dietel obtained 31 surgical liver biopsies during pregnancy and found only a slight increase in the number of binucleated liver cells when compared with 50 non-pregnant controls.

All these authors agree that histological liver changes during pregnancy are minor and nonspecific and that a "Schwangerschaftsleber" does not exist.

Liver blood flow

Liver blood flow is within the normal range in pregnancy. Using the bromsulfalein technic and hepatic vein catheterization Munnell and Taylor found a mean liver blood flow of 1,554 ml per minute per 1.73 sq.m. of body surface in 15 pregnant females (range 1,075—2,465) compared to a mean of 1,548 ml per minute (range 1,177—1,900) in 15 nonpregnant controls.

This is noteworthy because in pregnancy plasma volume and blood volume rise by 50 to 60 % and cardiac output increases by 30 to 50 % reaching a maximum in the 7th pregnancy month and returning to normal towards term. (Tysoe and Lowenstein.) Liver blood flow comprises 35 % of cardiac output in nonpregnant females and only 28 % of cardiac output in pregnancy. The excess blood volume is shunted through the placenta.

10

Hemoglobin and serum iron

Young et al. demonstrated a fall in hemoglobin levels during pregnancy in 219 serially examined patients. Hoch et al. found in addition a fall in serum iron levels, but could not demonstrate a correlation between hemoglobin and serum iron. In a more detailed study of 176 patients Niesert observed an average fall in hemoglobin from 95 % to 85 %, a fluctuating, but on the whole constant serum iron level, an increase in total iron binding capacity and a corresponding fall in iron saturation. Ikonen found the serum iron levels widely dispersed (range 59—294 microgm per 100 ml) in his 84 normal pregnancies.

Anemia during the last trimester of pregnancy is generally considered to be present only when the hemoglobin level falls to below 10 gm per 100 ml. The fall in hemoglobin and hematocrit is explained by the rise in plasma volume which is only partially compensated by a minor rise in red cell volume. (Tysoe and Lowenstein.)

Total leucocyte and differential count

Kuvin and Brecher found a normal white cell count and morphology in only 46 % of 88 pregnancies. 20 % have an increase of total white cells above 10,000 per cu. mm and counts of 15,000 per cu. mm are still considered normal in the last trimester. Abnormal differential counts are also common. There is an increase in both segmented and nonsegmented neutrophils. Not infrequently myelocytes and metamyelocytes may be seen which are not necessarily part of the "shift to the left".

Prothrombin time

The prothrombin time remains normal in all cases of uncomplicated pregnancy (Ikonen).

Urinary bile components

Although most textbooks state that urinary urobilinogen and urobilin may be increased in the later stages of pregnancy, few exact studies have been performed. Merletti in 1902 observed "as a rule" a two to three fold increase of urobilin in the last trimester. In normal pregnancies at term Arfwedson found "pathological bile components" in 5 % of 100 patients, Dieckmann et al. a positive urine bilirubin test in 14.5 % of 85 patients and Labo et al. a positive urine urobilin test in 8.3 % of 75 patients. On the other hand Cross reported bilirubin, urobilin and urobilinogen tests to be all normal in 61 uncomplicated pregnancies.

Serum bilirubin

Total serum bilirubin levels were reported to be normal during uncomplicated pregnancy by Cross in 61 patients, by Cantarow et al. in 34 patients, by Dieckmann et al. in 85 patients, by Wetstone et al. in 56 patients and by Thorling in 202 patients. The latter author gives a mean of 0.3 mg per 100 ml with a range of 0.1 to 1.1 mg per 100 ml.

Other authors report a mild serum bilirubin increase in a small percentage of normal pregnancies, e.g. Eufinger and Bader. Ikonen found bilirubin levels of 1.0 to 2.0 mg per 100 ml in 2 % of 100 patients, Arfwedson in 6 % of 100 patients and McNair and Jaynes in 4.3 % of 564 patients. Among Friedberg's 120 patients 15 % had a serum bilirubin of 1.0 to 1.5 mg per 100 ml and 1.7 % of more than 1.5 mg per 100 ml. Among Dieckmann et al.'s 85 patients with normal total bilirubin levels 20 % had an increase of the 1 minute direct-reacting fraction.

Neither Thorling nor McNair and Jaynes found a correlation between bilirubin levels and stage of gestation. There is no rise toward term, as does occur with alkaline phosphatase activity.

However, intravenous bilirubin tolerance tests are often impaired with advancing pregnancy. Among pregnant females with normal serum bilirubin levels Kaufmann found an increased bilirubin retention in 7 of 16 during the second half of pregnancy, Nürnberger in 13 of 25 toward the end of pregnancy, Soffer in 1 of 11 during the first trimester and in 9 of 10 during the second and third trimester, Sullivan et al. in 1 of 11 during the first half and in 15 of 47 during the second half of pregnancy. Soffer examined 10 patients twice and found in 7 a definite increase in bilirubin retention during the latter part of gestation. No studies of this nature have been performed since 1934.

Bromsulfalein retention

Normal bromsulfalein excretion during pregnancy was found in two early reports in 67 (Siegal) and 61 patients (Cross) except during labor. A slightly increased bromsulfalein retention was not infrequently reported towards term in later series. Thus, Christhilf and Bonsnes found a 5—10 % retention at 45 minutes in 6 of 36 and Cantarow et al. in 7 of 34 pregnancies at term. In the third trimester Labo et al. observed a 7—12 % retention in 7 of 75 pregnancies while Friedberg (1962) found a retention of more than 5 % in 11 % and of more than 10 % in 3.7 % of his patients. Mean bromsulfalein retention was reported by Wilken as 4 % during months 4—6, as 9.7 % during month 10 and as 16.3 % during labor. He ascribed this increased retention during labor to a temporarily reduced liver blood flow.

Combes et al., using the prolonged bromsulfalein infusion technique of Wheeler, found in 15 women in the second half of pregnancy a mean increase in relative hepatic storage capacity (S) of 122 % and a mean decrease of maximal excretory capacity (T_m) of 27 % while the results in the same women in the first half of pregnancy were no different from 10 normal nonpregnant controls. After delivery, T_m is normalized before S.

Galactose tolerance test

Urinary galactose excretion after an oral 40 g galactose load was found to be normal in 20 pregnancies at term by Nürnberger, while others claim it to be "often abnormal" (Friedberg 1960).

Serum alkaline phosphatase

Mean alkaline phosphatase activity rises slightly during the first half of pregnancy and then sharply during the seventh month, reaching a peak at term (Bodansky et al., Hoch et al., Speert et al.). Mean values obtained by different methods are given in Table 1. With different techniques the trend is the same but mean activites during the tenth

TABLE 1. Mean serum alkaline phosphatase activity during uncomplicated pregnancy

Alk. phosphatase method and units	Normal range	Month of gestation						Number of pat.	References
		5	6	7	8	9	10		
King-Armstrong	1 — 14	7.4	7.8	7.9	10.7	12.1	13.6	78	Mukherjee
Bodansky	1 — 4	—	2.9	3.2	3.6	4.7	5.9	300	Bodansky et al.
Buch & Buch	1 — 8	3.7	3.9	4.9	5.8	8.6	9.5	179	Thorling
Bessey-Lowry	0.8-2.3	1.4	1.6	1.7	2.3	3.1	2.7	43	Beck and Clark
Roberts	0 — 6	3.0	3.3	4.7	8.3	10.4	12.5	201	Meranze et al.
Vermehren	17 — 66	68	64	100	134	143	152	139	Vermehren
Shinowara-Jones-Reinhart	2 — 9	3.2	3.4	3.9	4.7	11.4	11.8	239	Friedman et al.

month differ markedly when compared to the respective upper limit of normal. The upper limit of normal is just reached with the King—Armstrong method. It is slightly surpassed in the Bodansky, Buch and Buch, Bessey—Lowry and the Shinowara—Jones—Reinhart technique and reaches twice the upper limit of normal with the Roberts and the Vermehren method. In individual women there may be little or no rise, in others the increase towards term is marked. (Thorling; Beck and Clark.) In the last two months 28 % surpassed 14 King—Armstrong units (Mukherjee), 4.1 % 20 King—Armstrong units (Young et al.), 11 % 5.5 Bessey—Lowry units (Ikonen), 60 % surpassed 4 and 20 % 6 Bodansky units (Bodansky et al.).

Alkaline phosphatase rises again during labor, especially in the second stage. In 15 serially examined women Mukherjee found mean alkaline phosphatases of 13.5 King—Armstrong units during the tenth month, 13.7 units during the first stage of labor, 18.2 units during the second stage of labor and 11.4 units on the 4th day after delivery. The underlying mechanism of this alkaline phosphatase rise is not clear. Generally it is felt to represent a physiological response to the demands made by the foetus during the last 3 months of gestation (Mukherjee). Beck and Clark believe that the excess phosphatase originates in the placenta. They found no increase of the alkaline phosphatase component which can be inhibited by sodium taurocholate and which is presumed to stem from bone and kidney. Alkaline phosphatase activity falls to pre-pregnancy levels within 4 to 6 weeks after delivery.

Serum transaminases and other serum enzymes

Serum glutamic oxalacetic transaminase remains normal throughout pregnancy (Mason and Wróblewski "extensive study", Borglin 34 cases, West and Zimmerman 70 cases, Knutson et al. 100 cases, Crisp et al. 30 cases, Stone et al. 71 cases, Kubli 32 cases, Friedman et al. 280 cases). Among Ikonen's 99 cases 96 were normal and 3 had SGOT levels between 40 and 80 units, all 3 being patients in labor. Mean SGOT levels during pregnancy are generally lower than in nonpregnant controls. Among West and Zimmerman's 70 cases none surpassed a value of 15 units during the first two trimesters. The means tend to rise toward term but remain within normal limits.

Serum glutamic pyruvic transaminase behaves identically (Rimbach and Bonow 25 cases, Ikonen 99 cases). Occasional elevations up to 80 units may be observed during labor.

Reports on *lactic dehydrogenase* during pregnancy are more conflicting. Normal values in all patients were reported by Linton and Miller (33 cases), Knutson et al. (100 cases), and Kubli (44 cases). West and Zimmerman report an increase in 2 out of 70 cases, but Hill in 19 out of 40 and Stone et al. in 9 out of 71 cases. During labor lactic dehydrogenase is elevated in nearly half the cases (West and Zimmerman 11 of 27, Kubli 13 of 35).

Serum ornithyl carbamyl transferase was slightly elevated in 7 of 46 normal pregnancies (Reichard et al.).

Serum cholinesterase activity diminishes progressively throughout pregnancy (Friedman et al.), Abnormally low values (less than 170 units) were found in 17 % of patients during the first trimester, in 33 % during the second trimester and in 43 % during the third trimester (Wetstone et al.).

Serum tributyrinase also shows a slight decrease in mean activity towards term (Friedman et al.).

Serum cholesterol and serum lipids

Serum cholesterol levels begin to rise in about the 4th pregnancy month and usually reach a maximum in the 8th month. McNair and Jaynes found values over 250 mg per 100 ml in 9 % of normal pregnancies in the 4th month, in 53 % in the 6th month and in 57 % in the 8th month. Similar findings were obtained by Wetstone et al. In the third trimester 6 of their 11 patients had serum cholesterol levels over 300 mg per 100 ml with a maximum of 435 mg per 100 ml. Serum cholesterol varied from 250 to 510 mg per 100 ml in 100 females with uncomplicated pregnancy near term reported by Ikonen, with the majority in the range of 300 to 420 mg per 100 ml. Von Studnitz, in a careful study of 101 females during the course of their pregnancy, found also an increase in total lipids, alpha lipoproteins, beta lipoproteins and phospholipids. These changes are presumed to be due to hormonal influence.

Total serum proteins and serum electrophoresis

Total serum protein levels fall gradually during pregnancy, reaching a low at term (Pfau, Wetstone et al., McNair and Jaynes). In a series of over 300 pregnant women McNair and Jaynes found serum protein levels below 6 gm per 100 ml in 7 % of patients during the 2nd pregnancy month and in 43 % during the 8th month. It must be remembered that during pregnancy circulating plasma volume increases by about 50—65 % and total body water by about 20 %.

In the detailed and serial observation of 21 women during their whole pregnancy by Coryell et al. total serum proteins declined by 13 % towards term. The albumin/globulin ratio fell from 1.32 before pregnancy to 1.21 in the second trimester, to 0.84 in the third trimester and to a low of 0.7 a few days after delivery. On electrophoresis there was a fall in albumin and gamma globulin and a rise in the alpha 1, alpha 2 and beta globulin fractions as well as in fibrinogen. These changes disappeared 6 to 12 weeks following delivery.

The erythrocyte sedimentation rate increases from the sixth month until term to about 30 mm per hour, Winthrobe (Tysoe and Lowenstein). This is probably related to the increase in fibrinogen.

Serum turbidity and flocculation tests

The reports regarding incidence of positive turbidity or flocculation tests during pregnancy are conflicting.

The *thymol turbidity* was normal in all of Thorling's 201 patients and in the 27 patients of Christhilf and Bonsnes. On the other hand, Labo et al. found 6.6 % abnormal reactions among 75 patients near term, Friedberg et al. 10.3 % among 120 patients, Ikonen in 12 % among 100 patients, McNair and Jaynes 6 % in early and 15 % in late pregnancy among some 300 patients and Dieckmann et al. 15 % positives in his 85 patients throughout pregnancy.

The *Takata-reaction* war normal in all of Thorling's 197 cases and positive in 20 % of Friedberg's 120 patients. The latter also found 20 % positive *cadmium-reactions.*

The *cephalin-flocculation test* was normal in all of Thorling's 197 and Christhilf and Bonsnes' 27 patients. Salmon found only 1 positive reaction in 71 patients. In contrast to these studies Labo et al. observed 6.6 % positive tests among 75 patients, McNair and Jaynes 8 % among 300 at term and Day and Hellestrand even 22.5 % of 101 patients.

It is possible that the test results are highly influenced by the specific technique and test reagents used in the different laboratories. Dieckmann et al. for instance reported in 1951 around 20 % positive cephalin flocculation tests among 85 women and even 40 % positives in the first trimester but 3 years later Dieckmann and Pottinger found only 5.2 % pathological reactions in 225 patients.

Conclusions

Of the many procedures used to evaluate "liver function" only the serum transaminases and the prothrombin time remain within normal limits in all pregnant women. Liver blood flow remains quantitatively unchanged while cardiac output increases. Liver histology may show minor and nonspecific changes, but is generally considered to be within normal limits.

There is an increased incidence towards term in spider naevi and palmar erythema. The following laboratory test results are often increased progressively with advancing pregnancy: total white cell count, number of segmented and non-segmented neutrophils, myelocytes and metamyelocytes, serum alkaline phosphatase, serum cholesterol, total serum lipids, bromsulfalein retention, hepatic bromsulfalein storage, serum alpha and beta globulins, fibrinogen and erythrocyte sedimentation rate.

An occasional increase not dependant on the stage of gestation is seen in serum bilirubin (up to 2 mg per 100 ml) and in the incidence of pathological serum turbidity and flocculation reactions. No careful studies exist on the incidence of pathological bile components in the urine. It is suggested that occasionally bilirubin, urobilin or increased amounts of urobilinogen may be present in uncomplicated pregnancy.

There is a decrease towards term in hemoglobin, erythrocyte count, hematocrit, total serum proteins, serum albumin, gamma globulin, serum cholinesterase, intravenous bilirubin tolerance and maximal bromsulfalein excretory capacity (T_m).

With the exception of total white cell counts most deviations from the normal are minor. The main diagnostic difficulties will be encountered with elevated alkaline phosphatase levels and pathological turbidity and flocculation tests. Determination of serum transaminases is the single most valuable test during pregnancy, although a normal result does not exclude the presence of liver disease.

II. Jaundice during pregnancy

1) Incidence of jaundice during pregnancy

Jaundice during pregnancy is rare. Table 2 is an attempt to summarize all reports in the literature from which incidence can be calculated. The overall figure is 557 cases of jaundice in 822,842 pregnancies, an incidence of 0.067 % or 7 cases per 10,000 pregnancies, or 1 case per 1,500 pregnancies. The total series has been subdivided in 2 parts: 10 reports which give "hepatitis" as only diagnosis, and 11 reports which list different etiologies including every case of jaundice during pregnancy. As can be seen, incidence of jaundice is slightly higher in the series which list "hepatitis" only. This does not make much sense. It may indicate that total incidence of jaundice during pregnancy reflects mainly the frequency of hepatitis during pregnancy in the respective series or that reports are mainly written after the experience of a hepatitis epidemic. Hepatitis accounts for at least 41 % of all cases with jaundice during pregnancy (see Table 4). This figure may in some areas during certain time periods approach 100 %.

In the single reports incidence of jaundice during pregnancy varies between 2 per 10,000 and 3 per 1,000 pregnancies, with the exception of 3 series collected during the height of a hepatitis epidemic. The highest observed incidence in reports covering more than a one year period is 8 hepatitis cases per 1,000 pregnancies (Zondek and Bromberg).

Excluding again series with observation periods of one year or less, the incidence of jaundice per year varies between 0.3 and 10.6 cases, with an average of 3 cases per year (415 cases in 138 years).

2) Classification of jaundice during pregnancy

The oldest classification of jaundice during pregnancy into "icterus levis" (those who survive) and "icterus gravis" (those who die) originates probably from Frerichs (1858) and is still used in the French literature with the addition of a third category, "ictère pseudo-grave" (those who look like they are going to die but eventually survive). Such a grouping is certainly clear-cut, but helpful to the clinician only in retrospect.

More meaningful is an attempt at an etiologic classification separating jaundice caused by pregnancy per se (only seen in pregnant women) from jaundice occurring by chance during the course of an otherwise uncomplicated gestation (seen also in non-pregnant females and in males). The classification given in

TABLE 2. Incidence of jaundice during pregnancy

Year	Authors	Country	Time period (years)	Total preg-nancies	Patients with jaundice	Incidence of jaundice in % of all pregn.	cases per year
Series with "hepatitis" as only diagnosis
1943	Saurer	Zürich	1	2,764	3	0.108	—
1947	Zondek & Bromberg	Jerusalem	9	12,360	3	0.024	0.3
	Zondek & Bromberg	Jerusalem	2.6	3,382	27*	0.798	10.1
1950	Dill	Washington D.C.	3	25,000	12	0.048	4.0
1951	Mickal	New Orleans	9	69,186	15	0.022	1.7
1953	Martini et al.	Hamburg	3.5	91,735	37	0.040	10.6
1955	Paul	Toronto	15	46,000	10	0.022	0.7
1956	Phatak & Patil	India	0.3	959	29	3.024	—
	Phatak & Patil	India	0.3	1,370	6	0.438	—
1957	Lacomme	Paris	?	10,000	10	0.100	—
1959	Mazaud et al.	Dakar	3	3,969	10	0.252	3.3
1959	Peretz et al.	Haifa	8	21,000	65	0.310	8.1
	Combined			287,725	227	0.078	
			53+		179+		3.4
Series with jaundice of different etiology
1951	Javert & Morrison	New York	?	74,087	51	0.069	—
1955	Thorling	Uppsala	10	25,797	72	0.279	7.2
1955	Meyer	Halle	1	1,550	18	1.161	—
1957	Vincent	New Orleans	17	136,179	32	0.023	1.9
1957	Enrile et al.	Philippines	7	14,944	7**	0.047	1.0
1961	Samuels	New Orleans	10	20,000	8	0.040	0.8
1962	Cahill	New York	28	110,378	52	0.047	1.8
1962	Synodinos et al.	Athens	6	44,000	37	0.084	6.2
1962	Cremona	Torino	2	9,870	6	0.061	3.0
1963	Siegler & Keyser	New York	(7-10)	80,356	25	0.031	—
1966	Haemmerli & Wyss	Zürich	5	17,956	22	0.122	4.4
	Combined			535,117	330	0.061	
			85+		236+		2.8
	Both collective series combined			822,842	557	0.067	
			138+		415+		3.0

* 29 cases in report, 2 with anicteric hepatitis have been excluded.

** 8 cases in report, 1 case of acute cholecystitis without jaundice is excluded.

+ Excluding series with collection periods of 1 year or less.

TABLE 3. Jaundice *during* pregnancy
        (Synonym: icterus gravidarum)

A. Jaundice *in* pregnancy
(Synonyms: icterus in graviditate, concommitant jaundice, coincidental jaundice, ictère intercurrent)

I. Usual forms of jaundice occurring also in non-pregnant subjects
    1. Hepatic parenchymal disease (especially viral hepatitis)
    2. Intrahepatic cholestasis (i.e. drug jaundice)
    3. Extrahepatic cholestasis (i.e. common duct stones)
    4. Congenital "idiopathic" hyperbilirubinemias
    5. Hemolytic disorders

II. Jaundice in typical medical complications of pregnancy
    1. Jaundice in severe pyelonephritis
    2. Jaundice in pyelonephritis and tetracycline toxicity
    3. Delayed chloroform poisoning
    4. Jaundice after (criminal) abortions
       (Clostridium perfringens septicemia, quinine toxicity etc.)

B. Jaundice *of* pregnancy
(Synonyms: icterus e graviditate, icterus graviditatis, icterus peculiar to pregnancy, ictère lié à la grossesse)

I. Idiopathic jaundice *of* pregnancy
    1. Intrahepatic cholestasis of pregnancy
       ("jaundice of late pregnancy", "recurrent jaundice of pregnancy")
    2. Acute fatty metamorphosis of pregnancy
       ("obstetric acute yellow atrophy")

II. Jaundice as a complication of another disease linked to pregnancy

    1. Jaundice in hyperemesis gravidarum
    2. Jaundice in vomiting of late pregnancy
    3. Jaundice in severe toxemia of pregnancy
    4. Jaundice in megaloblastic anemia of pregnancy
    5. Jaundice in hemolytic anemia of pregnancy

Table 3 seems to represent best our present state of knowledge.

Reviews of jaundice during pregnancy have been published by Mayer 1906, Kehrer 1907, Schickele 1910, Seitz 1916, Rissmann 1917, Eppinger 1923, Holmer 1927, Chabrol 1932, Eppinger 1937, Verhage 1940, Seitz 1948, Puyo 1953, Lichtman 1953, Dietel 1954, Caroli et al. 1954, Thorling 1955, Lacomme 1957, Brèt and Sénèze 1957 and 1958, Wilken 1958, Cattan and Cattan 1959, Dominici 1960, Richman 1960, Friedberg 1960, Labby 1960, Sheehan 1961, Meeroff 1961, Boquien et al. 1961, Cremona and Voghera 1962, Cahill 1962, Synodinos et al. 1962, Synodinos 1963, Friedberg 1963, Sherlock 1963, Ikonen 1964 and Gerl and Bonow 1964. The following reviews fail to mention recurrent jaundice of pregnancy (intrahepatic cholestasis of pregnancy): Winter 1890,

TABLE 4. Jaundice during pregnancy: Frequency distribution of different diseases in single reports

Year	Author	Total cases with jaundice	Hepatitis	Common duct stones	Hemolysis	Hyperemesis	Eclampsia	Cholestasis of pregnancy	Recurrent cholestasis of pregnancy	Other*	No diagnosis
1940	Verhage	43	6	2	1	15	14	—	1	4	—
1947	Nixon et al.	12	9	—	—	—	1	—	—	1	1
1951	Javert & Morrison	51	20	9	6	3	—	—	—	13	—
1955	Thorling	72	24	—	—	6	—	28	3	7	4
1955	Barry & O'Dwyer	9	5	—	—	—	1	1	—	2	—
1955	Meyer	18	8	1	1	3	3	—	2	—	—
1957	Vincent	32	25	2	—	—	—	—	—	5	—
1957	Enrile et al.	7	3	1	—	—	1	—	—	2	—
1961	Samuels	8	6	1	—	—	—	—	—	1	—
1962	Cahill	52	29	3	—	—	1	—	4	1	14
1962	Synodinos et al.	37	27	—	9	—	—	—	—	1	—
1962	Cremona	6	4	—	—	—	—	—	—	2	—
1963	Siegler & Keyser	25	12	2	1	—	—	1	—	5	4
1964	Ikonen	62	5	5	1	—	—	35	13	2	1
1966	Haemmerli & Wyss	22	6	1	—	—	—	—	6	—	9
	Combined series	456	189	27	19	27	21	65	29	46	33
	in %	100	41.5	5.9	4.2	5.9	4.6	14.2	6.4	10.1	7.2

* Detailed in table 5.

von Winckel 1893, Vinay 1894, Quirno et al. 1948, Lock et al. 1953, Puder 1955, Williams 1957, Millen 1957, Imparato 1958 and Varangot 1962. By far the most outstanding attempt at a clinical differential diagnosis is provided in Thorling's monography (1955).

3) **Frequency distribution of different diseases causing jaundice during pregnancy**

Fifteen reports, including 11 used in Table 2, break down their cases of jaundice during pregnancy into different etiologic categories. The 456 cases are summarized in tables 4 and 5. It is clearly evident, that infectious hepatitis constitutes the most frequent single disease entity. The figure of 41.5 % would be much higher, if the reports listing "hepatitis" as only diagnosis had been included. Many of these "hepatitis" reports exclude just a few cases of other etiologies, while some authors seem to feel that every case of jaundice during pregnancy is caused by viral hepatitis.

Table 4 lists the etiologic distribution reported by the individual authors.

TABLE 5. Jaundice during pregnancy: Frequency distribution of different diseases in 15 series combined (456 cases)

Diagnosis	Number of cases			%

Jaundice *in* pregnancy

1. Hepatocellular jaundice
   - Infectious hepatitis — 189
   - Acute yellow atrophy, non-specified [1] — 7
   - Cirrhosis [1],[2] — 4
   - Leptospirosis (Weil's disease) [3] — 1
   - Liver metastasis [2] — 1 } 212
   - Tuberculoma of liver [2] — 1
   - Echinococcus of liver [1],[4] — 2
   - Chlorpromazine jaundice [2],[5],[6],[7],[8] — 6
   - P.A.S. jaundice [8] — 1
2. Extrahepatic obstruction
   - Common duct stones — 27 } 28
   - Adenocarcinoma of common duct [3] — 1
3. Familial non-hemolytic jaundice [9] — 2 } 268 = 58.8
4. Hemolytic jaundice
   - Sickle cell anemia [4],[8] — 8
   - After blood transfusion [1] — 4
   - Hemoglobin H disease [4] — 1 } 19
   - Familial hemolysis (Spherocytosis) [4],[9] — 2
   - Not specified [1],[10] — 4
5. Mixed forms
   - Leukemia [1] — 2
   - Appendicitis with perforation [10] — 1
   - Infected cystadenoma of ovary [11] — 1 } 6
   - Septic shock [8] — 2

Jaundice due to complications of pregnancy
   - Hyperemesis gravidarum — 27
   - Eclampsia — 21
   - Marked hypertension without eclampsia [11] — 3
   - Severe pyelitis with jaundice [10],[11] — 5 } 60 = 13.9
   - After chloroform narcosis [12] — 1
   - After criminal abortion [2],[6],[10] — 3

Jaundice *of* pregnancy
   - Intrahepatic cholestasis of pregnancy — 65
   - Recurrent intrahepatic cholestasis of pregnancy — 29 } 96 = 21.0
   - Acute fatty metamorphosis of pregnancy [12],[13] — 2

No diagnosis — 33 = 7.2

456 = 100.0

References for table 5: [1] Javert & Morrison [2] Enrile et al. [3] Vincent [4] Synodinos et al. [5] Cahill [6] Cremona [7] Samuels [8] Siegler & Keyser [9] Ikonen [10] Verhage [11] Thorling [12] Barry & O'Dwyer [13] Nixon et al. References for unnumbered diagnosis are given in table 4.

These figures are in all likelyhood not accurate. They may reflect the trends in diagnosis by different clinicians and in different countries rather than actual incidence. For example, 63 out of the 65 cases of non-recurrent intrahepatic cholestasis of pregnancy are reported by two authors (Thorling and Ikonen). One case in our table is listed as "hepatitis" in the original report, but has been otherwise classified by us on the basis of the detailed published data (case 1 in Barry and O'Dwyer). It is very likely that many cases of intrahepatic cholestasis of pregnancy are hidden under the diagnosis "hepatitis", especially in series where this is the only diagnosis made. For instance 3 of 6 biopsies in Ingerslev's and Teilum's series of 91 "hepatitis" and 1 of 6 biopsies in the 65 "hepatitis" of Peretz et al. showed "normal" liver tissue, which is frequently seen in intrahepatic cholestasis of pregnancy. Intrahepatic cholestasis of pregnancy may possibly also be reported under jaundice due to choledocholithiasis, because the laboratory findings in both diseases may be identical. It is interesting in this regard, that 9 out of 27 cases with jaundice ascribed to common duct stones are contained in one single report. A rather interesting observation is that only 6 of the 15 reports admit to having cases of jaundice where no definite diagnosis could be reached.

Trends inherent in the time period during which the report was written may also influence the etiologic frequency distribution. Of course, no case of intrahepatic cholestasis of pregnancy will be reported before 1955, the year of Thorling's description of the disease. Cases of jaundice due to choledocholithiasis are few in single series after 1951, perhaps due to the more wide-spread use of cholangiography. More than half of the cases of jaundice second to hyperemesis or eclampsia are reported by a single author in 1940 (Verhage). It is possible that these disorders are better treated today and do less frequently progress to a jaundiced stage.

Geographic pathology also influences frequency distribution. Nine of 19 cases due to hemolytic jaundice are reported from Athens, due to the frequency of sickle cell anemia among the population admitted to that particular hospital. The same holds true for jaundice due to echinococcus of the liver.

Table 5 lists all diagnosis made in the 15 reports. It may serve as a survey of the rarer types of jaundice occasionally encountered. It is interesting to note, that among the 19 cases with hemolytic jaundice there is a conspicuous absence of "idiopathic hemolytic anemia of pregnancy" and of "pernicious anemia of pregnancy", two diseases quoted in most textbooks.

Few valid conclusions may be drawn from this type of survey. The diagnosis of "hepatitis" is probably made too often and on inconclusive evidence, but still viral hepatitis will account for the majority of cases with jaundice during pregnancy. Rarer than generally thought are obstructive jaundice due to common duct stones and hemolytic jaundice due to the state of gestation. Wrong diagnosis are probably made most often in cases of intrahepatic cholestasis of pregnancy, unless when recurrent in successive pregnancies.

TABLE 6. Incidence of viral hepatitis in relation to stage of gestation

Year	Authors	Cases of hepatitis			
		Total	1. Trim.	2. Trim.	3. Trim.
1951	Ingerslev & Teilum	88	2	1	85
1951	Javert & Morrison	20	5	2	13
1951	Mickal	15	0	4	11
1954	Ellegast et al.	52	14	21	17
1954	Frucht & Metcalfe	17	0	2	15
1955	Thorling	24	5	12	7
1955	Long, Boysen & Priest	10	1	3	6
1955	Hartmann & Schoen	26	6	10	10
1956	Ezès & Bourdon	34	2	25	7
1957	Dörfler	55	10	25	20
1959	Peretz et al.	65	7	25	33
1961	Denning & Bruckmann	21	7	4	10
1962	Cahill	29	8	6	15
	Total	456	67	140	249
	in %	100	14.7	30.7	54.6

4) Review of literature on jaundice during pregnancy

The following chapters are an attempt to summarize our present state of knowledge concerning the different forms of jaundice during pregnancy by a review of the available world literature.

Infectious hepatitis during pregnancy

The older literature and even some of the newer textbooks contain the following statements: pregnant women are especially susceptible to hepatitis; hepatitis in pregnant women occurs most frequently in the last trimester of pregnancy; hepatitis runs a severe course during pregnancy and results in a very high mortality. All these statements do not bear out under a critical evaluation of the literature.

Susceptability of pregnant women to viral hepatitis. The incidence of hepatitis in pregnant women runs parallel to epidemics in the general population. This is shown clearly in 5 reports. Zondeck and Bromberg in Jerusalem observed from 1934 to 1943 only 3 cases in 12,360 pregnancies, while in a 32 months period during 1943—1946 they saw 29 cases among 3,382 pregnancies. Peretz et al. reported 65 cases of hepatitis in Haifa during 1950 to 1957, 33 of which occured during 1950/1951. Ingerslev and Teilum in Copenhagen observed 15 cases during 1928 to 1940 and 91 cases during 1941 to 1949. Phatak and Patil in India reported in two successive 4 months periods 29 cases among

TABLE 7. Mortality from viral hepatitis during pregnancy

Country	Year of report	Author	Number of hepatitis	Number of deaths	Mortality %
Europe					
Zürich	1943	Saurer	3	0	0
Copenhagen	1951	Ingerslev & Teilum	91	1	1.1
Hamburg	1952	Dietel	8	2	25
Hamburg	1953	Martini, Harnack & Napp	57	1	1.7
Tübingen	1954	Schubert & Peters	26	1	3.8
Wien	1954	Ellegast et al.	69	1	1.4
Halle	1955	Meyer	8	0	0
Göttingen	1955	Hartmann & Schoen	26	0	0
Dublin	1955	Barry & O'Dwyer	7	0	0
Uppsala	1955	Thorling	24	0	0
Leipzig	1957	Dörfler	60	1	1.6
Bologna	1959	Labo, Facci & Raiti	41	1	2.5
Stuttgart	1961	Denning & Bruckmann	21	0	0
Zürich	1966	Haemmerli & Wyss	8	0	0
		Total	449	8	1.8
Mediterranean Area					
Istambul	1947	Nixon et al.	8	0	0
Jerusalem	1947	Zondek & Bromberg	27*	5	18.5
Tunis	1954	Corcos	8	4	50
Algiers	1956 / 1958	Ezès & Bourdon / Houel et al.	36	22	61.1
Cordoba	1957	Pirinoli	43	7	16.3
Haifa	1959	Peretz et al.	65	6	9.2
Dakar	1959	Mazaud, Moissinac & Labegorre	10	3	30.0
Athens	1962	Synodinos et al.	27	7	25.9
		Total	224	54	24.1
Asia					
India (Gwalior)	1956	Phatak & Patil	29	13	44.8
Philippines (Santo Thomas)	1957	Enrile et al.	3	3	100
		Total	32	16	50
North Amerika					
Maine	1947	Martin & Ferguson	4	0	0
New York	1951	Javert & Morrison	20	0	0
New Orleans	1951	Mickal	15	2	13.3
Boston	1952	Hsia, Taylor & Gellins	14	1	7.1
Boston	1952	O'Connell	2	0	0
Chelsea, Mass.	1953	Roth	16	0	0

Table 7. Cont.

Country	Year of report	Author	Number of hepatitis	Number of deaths	Mortality %
Boston	1954	Frucht & Metcalfe	17	2	11.7
Chicago	1955	Long, Boysen & Priest	10	2	25
Toronto	1955	Paul	10	0	0
New Orleans	1957	Vincent	25	6	24
Oregon	1960	Moore	2	1	50
New Orleans	1961	Samuels	6	0	0
New York	1962	Cahill	29	0	0
New York	1963	Siegler & Keyser	12	0	0
		Total	182	14	7.7
Combined series (38 reports)			887	92	10.4

* The report contains 29 cases. Two anicteric patients are excluded.

959 pregnancies and 9 cases among 1,370 pregnancies respectively. The most pertinent figures are provided by Martini, von Harnack and Napp. During a 42 months period in 1947 to 1950 they observed 37 hepatitis among 91,735 pregnancies. The population of Hamburg was 1,5 millions and 4,222 cases of hepatitis occurred during the same period. Among these were 270,000 women in the childbearing age group, 702 of which had hepatitis. The incidence of hepatitis is such 0.04 % among pregnant females, 0.07 % among women in the childbearing age group and 0.07 % in the general population.

A similar study from Vienna by Ellegast et al. (1954 b) reports the incidence of serum hepatitis in patients receiving intramuscular injections for the treatment of syphilis: 21.9 % in pregnant women (27 of 123), 20.6 % in nonpregnant females (156 of 759) and 21.1 % among males (168 of 796).

Pregnant women are thus clearly not more susceptible to the infection than the rest of the population. Saurer reports the case of a pregnant woman with hepatitis who infected 5 nurses connected with her immediate hospital care. These nurses in turn infected 6 of their roommates, while none of the other pregnant women on the ward got the disease.

Incidence of viral hepatitis in relation to stage of pregnancy. The reports giving the incidence of hepatitis in the various trimesters of pregnancy are collected in Table 6.

From this collective series there appears to be a definite increase of the incidence of hepatitis with advancing stage of pregnancy. Over half of the cases apparently occurred in the last trimester. Thorling has already pointed out that this type of statistics is fallacious. Most reported series were collected from obstetrical departments which are for obvious reasons largely composed of patients in the later stage of pregnancy. The series of Ingerslev and Teilum illustrates this best. Patients with hepatitis in the first trimester of pregnancy are more likely to be referred to other departments, as at this stage pregnancy itself does not yet take predominance in the handling of the patient. In most likelyhood hepatitis occurs with equal incidence in all trimesters of pregnancy, as is demonstrated in the two large series collected in departments of internal medicine (Ellegast et al., Dörfler).

Mortality from hepatitis during pregnancy. Table 7 gives the mortality figures for viral hepatitis during pregnancy collected from 38 reports in the literature. The overall figure of 92 deaths among 887 cases or 10.4 % appears markedly higher than the mortality in the general population from the same disease. A more meaningful interpretation of the data is achieved by dividing the reports geographically.

In Europe, a mortality of 1.8 % among 449 cases is certainly comparable to the usual mortality figures from hepatitis in the general population. Only one series shows a high mortality with 25 % or 2 out of 8 patients (Dietel). Here a selection of cases must play an important role, because Martini et al. report from the same town and from the same time period a series with 57 cases and a mortality of only 1.7 %.

In marked contrast to the low mortality in Europe is the high mortality in the Mediterranean area (24.1 %) and in Asia (50 %). The mortality is high in all series except the one from Istambul. This cannot be due to chance. An especially virulent virus in that area could be a possible explanation. Peretz et al. report that in Israel the new immigrants are not immunized to the middle East strain of hepatitis virus. More likely, the high mortality reflects the general debility and undernourishment of the indigene population. The 22 deaths from the series from Algiers occurred all in moslem women, who were brought to the hospital already in coma and died within hours to 4 days. In the report by Mazaud et al. from Dakar 3 of 6 African women died, but none of 4 European females. Zondek and Bromberg state that among their 27 patients 18 were definitely undernourished, including the 9 cases with a severe course. Their 5 deaths occurred in a 5 months period during the height of a virulent epidemic.

French authors often state that the combination of pregnancy and hepatitis has a very grave outlook. This view is readily understandable on the basis of the 3 reported French series: 29 of 54 patients died, a mortality of 53.7 %. However, these 3 series originate from Dakar, Tunis and Algiers, and no report on this topic has ever been published from the French mainland.

The series from the United States show an overall mortality of 7.7 %, but the single reports have either a very low or a very high mortality. This reflects probably the different hospital types in that country, admitting different population groups. In hospitals serving mainly people of the lowest income groups, undernourishment and general

TABLE 8. Clinical course in viral hepatitis during pregnancy

		Clinical course of hepatitis			
Author	Total cases	Mild	Moderate	Severe	Deaths
Schubert & Peters	26	17		9	1
Dörfler	60	29	29	2	1
Ellegast et al.	69	46	17	6	1

debility may play the same role as in the series from the Mediterranean area, and alcoholism could be an additional factor.

Clinical course of hepatitis during pregnancy. Statements regarding the clinical course of hepatitis during pregnancy by different authors vary according to the reported mortality in their series. Mortality, as we have already pointed out, depends mostly on the general condition of the patient material and not on the disease itself. The same geographic subdivision as for the mortality statistics seems indicated when discussing clinical course.

The severe cases from the Mediterranean area and Asia are not quite uniform. In the series of Ezès and Bourdon all 22 lethal cases were admitted in coma and died very rapidly, 7 of them even before delivery. Eleven delivered stillborn children and 4 premature living babies, 3 of which died shortly thereafter. Bilirubin levels in the mothers varied between 2.9 and 10 mg per 100 ml, alkaline phosphatases between 11 and 17 Bodansky units and blood urea nitrogen between 16 and 31 mg per 100 ml. Outstanding features were: very high white blood cell counts (25 to 30,000),

low blood sugars (between 14 and 40 mg per 100 ml in most) and very low prothrombin times (5 to 23 %). (Houel et al., same cases reported by different authors 3 years later). There was usually diffuse and massive bleeding from the gastrointestinal tract without obvious source at postmortem examination.

In the other series some of the comatous patients survived; 4 of 8 with coma reported by Corcos, 7 of 14 reported by Pirinoli, 5 of 16 reported by Phatak and Patil and 4 of 9 reported by Zondek and Bromberg. The latter authors stress as ominous signs the onset of tachycardia and a sudden drop in blood urea nitrogen, associated with a rise in serum amino acids and a slight rise in nonprotein nitrogen (to 38—40 mg per 100 ml). In the series from India serum bilirubin levels were strikingly low (2.0 to 6.6 mg per 100 ml).

Liver coma usually precipitates a spontaneous abortion. A spontaneous abortion in a severe case of hepatitis with or without coma does, however, not ameliorate the disease, in fact 3 of Corcos' patients developed lethal coma only a week after their abortion. Most authors agree today, that hepatitis in pregnancy is no indication for a therapeutic abortion.

27

In the reports from Europe, hepatitis during pregnancy is said to run a course no different from that in nonpregnant females or in males. In Martini et al.'s series bilirubin levels averaged 6.7 mg per 100 ml (range 0.7 to 24 mg per 100 ml). The only death occurred in a 38 year old woman with severe pyelonephritis. Thorling's 24 cases were all benign. Mean duration of hospitalisation was 24 days. Three authors classify their cases according to the severity of the clinical course (see Table 8).

Ellegast et al. compare the course in their 69 pregnant females with 360 nonpregnant hospitalised hepatitis cases. Mild forms were seen in 66.7 % of pregnant and 14.4 % of nonpregnant subjects, severe cases in 8.7 % of pregnant and in 15.8 % of nonpregnant patients. The 25 cases reported by Hartmann and Schoen were especially mild, with mean serum bilirubin levels of only 1.7 mg per 100 ml and an average hospitalisation of 19 days. Ingerslev and Teilum note also a high proportion of mild forms among their 91 patients. They further state that in 69 patients jaundiced up to the time of delivery the postpartum course was surprisingly uniform, in as much as jaundice cleared pretty regularly on the 11th post partum day, regardless of the duration of jaundice before delivery. This last feature is unusual for hepatitis during pregnancy and it is likely, that this series from Copenhagen includes many cases of intrahepatic cholestasis of pregnancy, which was still unknown in 1951. This assumption is supported by the fact that of their 6 liver biopsies only 3 showed hepatitis and the other 3 were "normal".

Furthermore, the thymol turbidity test was normal in the majority of cases.

It is possible that other series may be heavily weighed in favour of mild forms of hepatitis during pregnancy by undiagnosed cases of intrahepatic cholestasis of pregnancy. Still the conclusion appears valid, that the course of hepatitis — at least in Europe — is not influenced by pregnancy.

Pregnancy itself is influenced by hepatitis only by a tendency to premature delivery. Despite the often low prothrombin time in hepatitis uterine bleeding during delivery is very rarely marked, not even in patients in hepatic coma (Zondek and Bromberg). Ingerslev and Teilum note that 16 % of their 91 patients lost more than 500 ml blood during delivery, while 8 % appears to be the norm in their hospital. However, no case bled excessively.

Sequellae from hepatitis during pregnancy. Follow-up studies in women with hepatitis during pregnancy have been performed in 10 cases by Mickal, in 26 by Hartmann and Schoen and in 57 by Martini et al. No evidence of liver pathology was detected. Five of Martini et al.'s patients had subjective "liver symptoms" but were found to have completely normal liver functions.

The only disagreeing report is that of Frucht and Metcalfe, who re-examined 11 women and found only 2 "free of liver disease". One can hardly concur with this conclusion on the basis of their data. Five women had "enlarged livers", five had bilirubin levels of 1.0 to 1.8 mg per 100 ml and 4 had slightly increased globulin levels (in two of these deter-

TABLE 9. Fate of infants born from mothers with viral hepatitis

Author	Total cases of hepatitis	Spon-taneous abortions	Premature deliveries	Deaths of premature babies	Deaths in deliveries at term
Dietel	6	0	1	0	
Martini	54	2	11	0	
Ellegast et al.	47	0	16	4	2
Hartmann & Schoen	26	1	5	1	
Thorling	22	1	0	0	
Dörfler	55	3	10	1	
Denning & Bruckmann	19	1	2	0	
Total Europe	229	8	45	6	2
Zondek & Bromberg	29	0	7	0	
Pirinoli	37	1	16	9	
Synodinos et al.	20	0	1	1	1
Total Mediterranean	86	1	24	10	1
Mickal	13	0	1	1	
Roth	16	2	0	0	1
Paul	10	0	5	3	
Cahill	29	2	3	1	
Total North America	68	4	9	5	1
Total combined series	383	13	78	21	4
in %	100	3.4	20.4	5.5	1.0

mined during a new pregnancy). However, bromsulfalein excretion and flocculation tests were normal in all. Similarly, Ley and Liebl examined 42 women 2 to 8 years after their pregnancy with hepatitis. They found minor chemical abnormalities in this group (thymol turbidity 2 + in 30 %, Takata reaction slightly positive in 10 % and borderline bilirubin elevation in 2 cases), but there was no difference when compared to a similar follow-up study in 69 cases with hepatitis outside pregnancy. One case only had chemical evidence of probable mild liver disease. Zondek and Brom-

berg are the only authors to report 2 cases of chronic hepatitis among their 23 survivors.

Thus, incidence of residual liver disease after hepatitis during pregnancy is certainly not more frequent than in patients with hepatitis outside of pregnancy.

Child survival from mothers with hepatitis during pregnancy. Hepatitis during pregnancy induces a tendency toward abortion or premature delivery, as does any other form of jaundice. The mechanism is unknown. There is no correlation between premature delivery and duration of jaundice, serum bilirubin level or severity of clinical course. (Ellegast 1954 a.) Survival of the babies depends on their stage of maturity at birth and not on the mother's disease. Table 9 summarizes the available data from the literature, excluding cases with therapeutic abortions.

In the combined series of 383 cases 9.9 % of the babies died: 3.4 % abortions, 5.5 % prematures and 1.0 % of babies delivered at term. There were 20.4 % premature deliveries (19.6 % in the European and 27.9 % in the Mediterranean series). Of all prematures 13.6 % died in the European and 41.7 % in the Mediterranean collective series.

Harnack and Martini report 20 women who had hepatitis 1 to 7 months before conception and were not jaundiced during pregnancy. There were 2 abortions and 1 premature delivery in this series.

A follow-up study in children born of mothers with infectious hepatitis is reported by Ellegast et al. (1954 c). Only 1 child was transiently jaundiced on the 7th day for 1 week, the others did not show any evidence of liver disease.

Transplacentar infection with hepatitis virus and incidence of malformation in babies of mothers with hepatitis during pregnancy. The problem of transplacentar infection of the embryo or baby with the hepatitis virus has been extensively discussed by several authors (Stokes et al., von Harnack and Martini, Ellegast et al. 1954 c, Mansell, Dörfler 1957 and Dörfler 1958). The evidence for its occurrence is very meager.

Hepatitis in babies within their first two months of life does occur, but their mothers are but exceptionally jaundiced during pregnancy. On the other hand, practically none of the babies of mothers with clear-cut hepatitis during pregnancy have hepatitis. Ellegast et al. theorise that the babies are protected by the antibodies of their mothers, and that infection would only occur when viremia in the mother is present shortly before delivery, i.e. before the formation of antibodies.

Dörfler in 1958 collected the available reports on the incidence of malformations. Among 528 cases of hepatitis during pregnancy he found 19 malformations (reported in Harnack and Martini, Ellegast et al. 1954 c, Bickenbach, Mansell). This incidence of 3.5 % is not significantly different from the "normally" expected malformation rate of 2.4 %. Not included in Dörfler's review are 2 malformations reported by Ingerslev and Teilum and 1 case reported by Cahill, all 3 with hepatitis in the second half of pregnancy. Most of these mothers were ill with hepatitis during the last trimester of gestation, which would not account for the malformations in their babies. Kellog and Wesp observed a woman with hepatitis one month before conception who then delivered a monster. A causal relationship is possible in this case.

Thus, transplacentar infection with hepatitis virus and malformation of babies has not been completely ruled out, but — if it does occur — appears to be extremely rare.

Jaundice in liver cirrhosis during pregnancy

Cirrhosis of the liver and pregnancy is a very rare coincidence. Most cases of cirrhosis in women are seen past the childbearing age (Burslem et al.). In young women with cirrhosis fertilisation is frequently precluded by the high incidence of amenorrhoea, oligomenorrhoea and non-ovulatory cycling (Labby).

At least 31 patients with cirrhosis of the liver and pregnancy are reported in the literature (Scaglione 1923, Kraul 1927, Hesseltine 1930, Tenney and King 1933, Ashton 1934, Lascano and Pereyra 1936, Javert and Morrison 1951 3 cases, Burslem et al. 1952 2 cases, Puyo 1953 2 cases, Mack et al. 1953 2 cases, Slater 1954, Bearn et al. 1956 2 cases, Abrams 1956, Enrile et al. 1957, Adno 1957, Nabriski et al. 1958 2 cases, Labby 1960, Moore and Hughes 1960 3 cases, O'Leary and Bepko 1962, Bennet et al. 1963, Slaughter and Krantz 1963 2 cases). The age ranges from 23 to 42 years in these patients. Five underwent 2 pregnancies after cirrhosis had been documented (Burslem et al. case 2, Abrams, Nabriski et al. case 2, Moore and Hughes case 3, Slaughter and Krantz case 1).

Not all cases are reported with enough details to allow for an exact tabulation. In at least 10 of the 31 patients there were no signs of deterioration of liver function during pregnancy (Kraul, Tenney and King, Burslem et al. both cases, Bearn et al. both cases, Adno, Nabriski et al. case 2, Moore and Hughes case 1, Slaughter and Krantz case 2). An 11th case had no symptoms during the course of gestation and massive, but controllable uterine bleeding during delivery (Ashton). At least 7 of these 11 patients had jaundice, ascites and/or hematemesis prior to the reported asymptomatic gestation.

One patient developed ascites during pregnancy (Abrams) and in another pre-existing ascites increased (Hesseltine). A total of 8 patients were jaundiced during pregnancy. In 4 pre-existing jaundice became more intense (Slater, Labby, Moore and Hughes cases 2 and 3) and in 3 jaundice developed during the last trimester of pregnancy. In 2 of these jaundice persisted for several months post partum (Puyo) and the third patient died 5 days after delivery in hepatic coma (Enrile et al.). In the 8th patient jaundice decreased towards term (Bennet et al.).

Only 4 patients developed hematemesis during pregnancy. In one it started in the 20th week of gestation, could not be controlled and the patient died (Lascano and Pereyra). In a second case hematemesis occurred during the 5th month and was successfully stopped by performing a porto-caval shunt (O'Leary and Bepko). The third case had hematemesis near term and ceased to bleed after a Caesarian section (Nabriski et al. case 1). In the 4th case hematemesis started during labor and the patient exsanguinated (Scaglione).

There are a total of 4 deaths attributable to a complication of cirrhosis during pregnancy: 2 are due to hematemesis (in 1923 and 1936), 1 due to hepatic coma, and a fourth case report gives no details (Javert and Morrison). In addition there were 2 late deaths: 1 six months post partum from the sequellae of a splenectomy (Ashton) and 1 a year after delivery from liver failure (Slater).

Only 5 of the 36 children in this series died: 2 still-births in the 20th week (Lascano and Pereyra) and near term (Bennet et al.), 1 of congenital abnormalities (Moore and Hughes case 3) and 2 during delivery (Mack et al. case 2, Slaughter and Krantz case 1).

Five patients had porto-systemic shunts performed prior to the reported pregnancy: 2 porto-caval shunts (Bearn et al. case 24, Abrams) and 3 spleno-renal shunts (Adno, Labby, Slaughter and Krantz case 2). In all 5 there were no complications during gestation.

In addition to these 31 patients with Laennec's or postnecrotic cirrhosis 3 pregnant patients with primary biliary cirrhosis are reported by Ahrens et al. They suffered no ill effect from pregnancy.

In general therefore, pregnancy is surprisingly well tolerated in a woman with cirrhosis of the liver. It is probable that patients with the more severe forms of cirrhosis do not become pregnant and that the majority of cirrhotics with pregnancy represent a selection of benign cases.

Drug-induced intrahepatic cholestasis during pregnancy

Of the long list of drugs capable of producing intrahepatic cholestasis (Dölle and Martini) *chlorpromazine* is the one most frequently used during pregnancy. It has been advocated for the treatment of hyperemesis gravidarum by Moyer et al. and by Benaron et al. No cases of jaundice occurred in their 78 and 158 pregnancies respectively. In the series of Stacey et al. 8 of 170 non-pregnant patients (4.8 %) developed icterus. Love and Peel collected 10 single case reports of chlorpromazine jaundice during pregnancy.

Chlorpromazine jaundice during pregnancy, whether short-lasting or chronic, has no ill effect on the child. Clinically it may simulate intrahepatic cholestasis of pregnancy during the icteric stage. It usually starts much earlier because the drug is given for hyperemesis during the first trimester and usually clears well before delivery. Onset of chlorpromazine jaundice is within 4 weeks after the drug has been started. There is a prodromal phase of 4 to 5 days' duration, usually acute, with malaise, fever, chills, nausea, mild abdominal pains, myalgias and occasionally skin rashes. Itching may precede jaundice (Werther and Korelitz, Sherlock). These prodromal symptoms are similar to those seen in viral hepatitis and will readily distinguish drug-induced cholestasis from intrahepatic cholestasis of pregnancy, in which there are no prodromi except pruritus.

On occasion chlorpromazine jaundice may become chronic, and the question whether pregnancy may induce chronicity is unsettled. Read et al. collected 22 cases with chlorpromazine jaundice of more than 3 months' duration. Three of these started during pregnancy and include the case with the longest duration on record, i.e. 3 years. This woman (case 1 of Read et al.) was given chlorpromazine 75 mg daily during 8 days for hyperemesis and developed intrahepatic cholestasis with a maximum serum bilirubin of 21.6 mg per 100 ml, an alkaline phosphatase of 256 King—Armstrong units and a serum cholesterol of 1,120 mg per 100 ml. Later xanthomatosis appeared and the clinical picture resembled primary biliary cirrhosis. The jaundice cleared after 3 years and the xanthomas were fading after 4 years. A case of 10 months' duration is recorded by Gebhardt et al. and one of 7 months' duration by Stacey et al. A fourth case of chronic chlorpromazine jaundice starting during pregnancy (not contained in Read's et al.'s review) is reported by Love and Peel, with a duration of 6 months. All patients recovered completely. The longest duration of icterus in non-pregnant subjects has been 9 and 13 months, with jaundice of less than 7 months' duration in all the others.

Drug-induced intrahepatic cholestasis, clinically and histologically of the chlorpromazine type, has also been described after *nitrofurantoin* (Furodantin®) in an elderly female (Ernaelsteen and Williams) and recently in a pregnant woman (Goldstein and Contino). In both instances pyelonephritis for which the drug was given was severe but responded rapidly to treatment, whereas jaundice persisted for some weeks.

Obstructive jaundice due to choledocholithiasis during pregnancy

Jaundice due to common duct obstruction by gallstones is rare during pregnancy. In our collective series on jaundice during pregnancy there are only 27 cases recorded (table 4). Nine of these are contained in a single paper, which casts some doubt on the diagnostic accuracy. The rarity of this association even provokes single case reports (Rissmann 1909 and 1910, Brocq et al., Alex).

Gallstones have been said to occur more frequently in women with previous pregnancies than in childless women (Horn). Potter noted large atonic gallbladders with thick, tarry and viscous bile in three fourth of 390 women undergoing Caesarian sections. However, this did not cause stone formation. Large et al. examined 352 pregnant women with cholecystographies and found gallstones in only 11. Furthermore, a large collective autopsy statistic by Robertson and Dochat showed that of 14,016 women with gallstones at autopsy 79.6 % had been previously pregnant but the incidence of previous pregnancies was nearly identical (79.2 %) in autopsies of females without gallstones.

Jaundice during pregnancy due to an adenocarcinoma of the common duct has been noted twice (Caroli et al. 1954, Vincent).

Effect of pregnancy in chronic idiopathic hyperbilirubinemias (Dubin—Johnson syndrome, Roter syndrome, Gilbert—Meulengracht syndrome)

In a review in 1958 Dubin collected 53 cases of chronic idiopathic jaundice *(Dubin—Johnson syndrome)*. Nine of the 53 were women and 7 of the 9 underwent one or several pregnancies. (Dubin 1958 cases 16, 18 and 22, Klayman and Efrati, John and Knudtson, Tamaki, Carfagno). Pregnancy had no effect on the clinical course in one case, precipitated an attack of jaundice in 2 and aggravated pre-existing jaundice in 4. Icterus became gradually more intense, reached its height in the third trimester and waned or disappeared completely after delivery of the child. Clinically the disease may simulate extrahepatic biliary obstruction, but itching is absent and the alkaline phosphatase is usually within normal limits. Diagnosis may be suspected from the history of chronic jaundice without severe impairment of health and is easily verified by liver biopsy.

A similar syndrome but with normal liver biopsy findings has been described by Rotor. It is not clear at present, whether this is a disorder by itself or a milder form of the Dubin—Johnson syndrome. The patients with the *Rotor syndrome* have permanent mild jaundice but are otherwise asymptomatic. One woman reported in the literature underwent three pregnancies, each time with a decrease in the intensity of jaundice (Haverback and Wirtschafter, case 2).

In both the Rotor and the Dubin—Johnson syndrome the direct-reacting serum bilirubin fraction is elevated. A normal direct-reacting bilirubin with a mild elevation of the indirect-reacting fraction occurs in the *Gilbert—Meulengracht syndrome*. These patients are asymptomatic except for some fatigue (Foulk et al.). The syndrome occurs less frequently in females than in males. Stress, exercise and upper respiratory infections are said to increase jaundice temporarily. The effect of pregnancy on bilirubin levels in these patients has not been studied. Meulengracht reports two women who were free of jaundice during gestation.

Hemolytic jaundice during pregnancy
Hemolytic jaundice during pregnancy is very rare (Zachariae). It may be observed after incompatible blood transfusions. Jaundice observed in severe eclampsia and in overwhelming infections (pyelonephritis) has been classified by Sheehan as hemolytic.

Megaloblastic anemia of pregnancy may cause severe anemia, but rarely visible jaundice. In most cases it is due to dietary folic acid deficiency (Sanders). Occasionally vitamin B_{12} deficiency may be encountered, but is, if present, usually combined with folic acid deficiency (Lowenstein et al.). *Hemolytic anemia of pregnancy* (without demonstrable cause other than pregnancy itself) may produce jaundice, but is extremely rare (Dameshek and Schwartz, Crismer).

More often, hemolytic jaundice during pregnancy is caused by an exacerbation of a pre-existing chronic hemolytic state (Bromberg et al.). This may occur in congenital spherocytosis (Rimbach and Beickert) and in some hemoglobinopathies, especially in S—C, S—S and C—C disease (Fouché and Switzer, Curtis). Jaundice may become marked in some instances. The combination of gestation and hemoglobinopathy is hazardous for both mother and child.

A rare case may have a combined etiology, such as megaloblastic anemia of pregnancy superimposed on congenital spherocytosis (Schneider and Frahm).

A classification of hemolytic anemias during pregnancy is given in the paper of Zachariae.

During pregnancy hemolysis presents as marked anemia and an accompanying hemolytic jaundice will practically never pose a diagnostic problem.

Rare causes of jaundice during pregnancy

Of course, any disease capable of producing jaundice may once in a while be encountered during pregnancy, such as echinococcus of the liver (Javert and Morrison, Synodinos et al.), tuberculoma of the liver (Enrile et al.), Weil's disease (Vincent), diffuse liver metastasis (Vincent) and leukemia (Javert and Morrison). A differential diagnosis of jaundice per se is beyond the scope of this paper.

Jaundice in severe pyelonephritis during pregnancy

Before the advent of antibiotics pyelonephritis with jaundice was not infrequently seen during pregnancy (Decaudin). Jaundice was probably due to overwhelming septicemia. Toxic hemolysis may play an additional role (Rimbach).

Lepage, in his thesis in 1934, collected 27 cases from the literature and added 4 of his own, calling the syndrome "pyélonéphrite dite gravido-toxique". In our collected series from the literature since 1940 only 5 of 456 cases of jaundice during pregnancy were due to pyelonephritis (Table 5). Sheehan's autopsy series contains 12 pregnant women dying from pyelonephritis, 3 of which had mild jaundice during the last few days of life. The livers showed only mild nonspecific changes.

This entity has now become rare. Pyelonephritis can be treated today before it progresses to a jaundiced stage. Effective treatment of pyelonephritis during pregnancy has, however, created a new hazard: jaundice in pyelonephritis of pregnant women due to drug toxicity (see next paragraph).

Jaundice during pregnancy due to toxicity of drugs used in treatment of pyelonephritis (Tetracycline toxicity).

Schultz et al. reported 6 autopsy cases of pregnant women treated for pyelonephritis with extremely high dosis of intravenous tetracycline (2.4 to 4.0 gm per day). The patients became jaundiced 3 to 5 days after treatment was started, with bilirubin levels of 5 to 12 mg per 100 ml, alkaline phosphatase of 9 to 44 King—Armstrong units, positive cephalin flocculations and mild elevation of serum glutamic oxalacetic transaminases (70—170 units). The patients died within 5 to 13 days. The livers showed diffuse fatty metamorphosis.

One of the two cases reported by Kahil et al. and the case of Lewis et al. both diagnosed as acute fatty metamorphosis of pregnancy, had also received high dosis of tetracycline and streptomycin for severe pyelonephritis. At post-mortem examination fatty metamorphosis was diffuse and the characteristic rim of intact liver cells in the periphery of all lobules seen in acute fatty metamorphosis of pregnancy was not present.

Whalley et al. reported 5 similar cases with survival in four. Their treatment for pyelonephritis consisted of intravenous tetracycline, 1.5—2 gm per day and intramuscular streptomycin 1 gm per day for 4—17 days. All had renal failure and an associated pancreatitis. Fatty metamorphosis was predominantly centrolobular in the liver biopsies of the 4 survivors and diffuse in the post mortem examination. Necrosis and inflammation were absent. Serum bilirubin ranged from 3.5 to 18.8 mg per 100 ml, alkaline phosphatase from 8 to 29 Bodansky units, SGOT from 34 to 650 units and thymol turbidity and cephalin flocculation were positive. Blood urea nitrogen was elevated to between 40 and 130 mg per 100 ml and serum amylase to between 580 and 3,200 units. Serum levels of tetracycline were 38 and 63 micrograms per ml in 2 cases 1 week after tetracycline treatment was stopped (normal therapeutic levels 1 to 5 micrograms per ml).

This observation implicates tetracycline as the responsible toxic agent. It is curious that this type of tetracycline toxicity has never been observed outside pregnancy and that the liver lesion is nearly indistinguishable from acute fatty metamorphosis of pregnancy, which does also not occur outside of gestation.

Nitrofurantoin (Furodantin®)-induced intrahepatic cholestasis is another but benign disorder occurring in the treatment of pyelonephritis. It occurs also in non-pregnant subjects and has been discussed in the chapter on drug-induced cholestasis.

Jaundice due to delayed chloroform poisoning
This form of jaundice occurs only after delivery and is furthermore mainly of historic interest. It shall be mentioned here because it rarely occurred in non-obstetric patients.

Sheehan reported 14 autopsy cases in 1940, which fell into 3 groups. Three patients apparently healthy aside from pregnancy had received an overdose of chloroform and died within 2 days without evidence of hepatic dysfunction. At autopsy there were isolated cell lesions involving more than half of the hepatocytes in the middle and center of the lobules. Nine patients with prolonged labor before chloroform narcosis developed jaundice, fever and coma on the second postpartum day and died 2 to 4 days later. The striking finding at autopsy was a band of mid-zonal necrosis. Two patients with severe hyperemesis before chloroform narcosis had central necrosis at postmortem examination.

Intrahepatic cholestasis of pregnancy
Intrahepatic cholestasis of pregnancy is — after viral hepatitis — the second most frequent cause of jaundice during pregnancy. It accounts for 20.6 % of the 456 cases with jaundice listed in Table 4. It has a marked tendency to recur in subsequent pregnancies, but is entirely benign to both mother and child. The disease is characterized by marked pruritus followed by mild jaundice with no other prodromal symptoms and no impairment of general well-being. Jaundice appears in the majority of cases after the 22nd week of gestation, but may start as early as the 7th week in some patients. Jaundice and pruritus disappear rapidly after spontaneous or induced delivery. Biochemically the disorder presents the features of "obstructive jaundice" with no evidence of parenchymal liver cell damage. Bile flow in the extrahepatic biliary passages is unimpaired. Liver biopsies show minimal intrahepatic cholestasis.

Details on clinical, biochemical and

histological features of this disease will be discussed in the chapter on recurrent intrahepatic cholestasis of pregnancy.

Acute fatty metamorphosis of pregnancy
In 1940 Sheehan delineated from true acute yellow atrophy of the liver due to fulminating viral hepatitis a new entity "obstetric acute yellow atrophy", which was later termed "acute fatty metamorphosis of pregnancy" by Ober and Lecompte. Its etiology is unknown, but it occurs only in pregnant females. This entity presents a clear-cut and diagnostic histological picture of the liver, but is clinically nearly indistinguishable from fulminant viral hepatitis.

Histologically it consists of a gross fatty change which starts in the center of the acini and involves finally the entire liver lobule with the exception of a sharply defined rim of normal liver cells around the portal tracts. There is a striking absence of necrosis and of inflammatory reaction. Only occasionally a very light infiltration of small round cells may be seen throughout the fatty area. The portal tracts show no abnormalities (Sheehan 1940). Bile thrombi may be present in the center of the lobules (Moore). Compared to fulminant hepatitis there is a striking lack of postmortem autolysis. In the one survivor followed by serial liver biopsies (Whitacre and Fang) restitution of liver cells began from the remaining rim of normal cells in the periphery of the lobules and then progressed towards their center.

Some confusion exists in the literature resulting from the inclusion of cases with diffuse fatty metamorphosis without a peripheral rim of intact liver cells. Such cases probably do not belong to the entity described by Sheehan. The case reported by Lewis et al. for instance is a typical example of tetracycline toxicity in pyelonephritis during pregnancy. Tetracycline toxicity must be implicated also in case 1 reported by Kahil et al.

In the literature 40 cases of acute fatty metamorphosis of pregnancy have been reported (Stander and Cadden 1934, Cullinan 1936 cases A and B, Sheehan 1940 6 cases, Whitacre and Fang 1942, Nixon et al. 1947 case 20, Barry and O'Dwyer 1955 case 9, Ober and Lecompte 1955 3 cases, Moore 1955, Moore 1956 4 cases, Mason 1958, Dyson 1959, Nardone et al. 1961, Sheehan 1961 2 cases, Bruno and Ober 1962 5 cases, Peters et al. 1963 7 cases, clinicopathologic conference 1963, Siegler and Keyser 1963, Kahil et al. 1964 case 2). Not included in this review are 11 additional cases: 6 because the histological findings are different or inconclusive (Baens and Espinola 1937, Dill 1950 cases 1, 2 and 6, Lewis et al. 1963, Kahil et al. 1964 case 1) and 5 in which the patients recovered and no liver biopsies were performed (Duncan and McLachlan 1933, Taylor 1952, Pirinoli 1957, Edwards 1960, Sheehan 1961).

Acute fatty metamorphosis of pregnancy has been noted in the age range of 16 (Ober and Lecompte case 3) to 42 years (Nardone et al., Dyson). In the majority of cases it occurred during the first pregnancy. In only 3 of 40 cases it was observed after the second gestation: during the third pregnancy in the CPC case, during the sixth in Moore's case 2 and during the 8th in case 2 of Nardone et al.

Onset of symptoms was in 30th week in two cases (Moore case 1 and 2), in the 31st week in 1 (Ober and Lecompte case 1), in the 34th in 2 (Moore case 4, CPC case) and in the others between the 36th and 40th week. The disease starts rather suddenly with severe and persistent vomiting, occasionally accompanied by abdominal pains, followed in a few days by jaundice. Tachycardia of between 100 and 130 is regularly present, but there is no fever. The symptoms then progress rapidly, the jaundice becomes intense, the patient somnolent, the vomiting assumes a coffee-ground aspect and frank hematemesis may supervene. Severe headaches are noted in some patients. The laboratory features are consistent with an obstructive jaundice, except that urinary bilirubin may not be present until terminally. The highest recorded serum bilirubin levels were 12.7 (Whitacre and Fang), 16.8 (Moore case 3) and 26 mg (CPC case) per 100 ml, all others being below 10 mg per 100 ml. The alkaline phosphatase is increased to levels up to 54 King—Armstrong units (Moore). Serum transaminases have been recorded in only 2 cases with values between 100 and 300 units (CPC, Kahil et al.). Thymol turbidity and cephalin flocculation tests are normal with one exception (Kahil et al.). Prothrombin time is markedly decreased. White cell counts ranged from 19,200 to 32,000 per cu. mm. in the 7 recorded cases (Barry and O'Dwyer, Ober and Lecompte, Kahil et al., CPC). A few patients had marked hypoglycemic episodes (Stander and Cadden, Whitacre and Fang, Kahil et al.). In about half of the cases oliguria sets in, followed by azotemia. A disproportionate rise of uric acid levels has been noted by Sheehan, and a disproportionate rise of serum creatinine in the CPC case. Others have seen a drop of the previously elevated blood urea nitrogen to abnormally low levels just before death (Barry and O'Dwyer, Mason, CPC).

The usual course is steadily downhill. Premature labor sets in, the woman delivers a stillborn child and then lapses into deep coma, occasionally accompanied by convulsions. High fevers may now occur and the patient dies shortly thereafter. The duration from the first symptom until death may vary between 3 days and 4 weeks and is usually between 1 and 2 weeks. The duration from delivery to death is usually 2 to 4 days, but may range from one hour (Ober and Lecompte case 3) to a maximum of 7 days (Moore case 4).

Some minor exceptions to this typical course may occur. Two cases died undelivered before ever having been jaundiced (Dyson, Nardone et al.), another died undelivered during the icteric stage (Cullinan, case A). In 2 others the first symptom appeared only after delivery (case 20 of Nixon et al., case 3 of Moore) and in one jaundice began 4 days post partum (Ober and Lecompte, case 2). In two cases pruritus was present (Ober and Lecompte case 1, CPC case). Four patients developed ascites (Ober and Lecompte case 1, Moore case 3, Whitacre and Fang, Kahil et al. case 2). Two patients bled profusely during delivery (Mason, CPC case). At autopsy a clinically unsuspected acute hemorrhagic pancreatitis was found in 3 of Bruno and Ober's and in 4 of Peters et al.'s cases. Fatty degeneration of the renal tubules was noted in 7 cases on postmortem examination (Ober and Lecompte 3 cases, Dyson, Nardone et al., Sheehan 1961, CPC). Associated preeclampsia was present in 5 patients (Nixon et al., Dyson, Sheehan 1940, Nardone et al., Kahil et al.).

Of the 40 acceptable cases only 6 women survived. Two of these are reported in abstract form (Peters et al.) and in a third no details are given (Siegler and Keyser). Of the remaining 3 cases 2 were delivered by an early Caesarian section (Whitacre and Fang, Moore case 2) and in one the first symptom occurred after delivery (Moore case 3). Another 5 cases with recovery but without histological proof of the diagnosis have been mentioned above.

Only 5 children survived in the 40 acceptable cases: one in a case with onset of symptoms after delivery (Nixon et al.), the two children delivered by Caesarian section from which the mothers survived also (Whitacre and Fang, Moore case 2) and two after spontaneous delivery (Stander and Cadden, Ober and Lecompte case 1).

Acute fatty metamorphosis of pregnancy is thus a rare, but distinct entity not occurring outside of pregnancy. It carries a grave prognostic outlook, but is potentially reversible. As rapid deterioration sets in always after delivery and as both women delivered by Caesarian section survived, it appears reasonable to propose as an only chance for both mother and child a therapeutic Caesarian section as early as possible after onset of symptoms.

Jaundice in hyperemesis gravidarum

Jaundice in hyperemesis gravidarum is rare, usually mild and does not imply a poor prognostic outlook. In a thesis in 1926 Ferru could collect only 22 cases from the literature, one of which died.

Of 51 patients with hyperemesis reported by Verhage 15 had a slight serum bilirubin elevation, but only a few were frankly jaundiced. Urinary urobilinogen was increased in most and urine bilirubin was present in about one third. Of Millar's 120 patients 5 were jaundiced. In Klier's series of 119 patients 12 had elevated serum bilirubin levels ranging from 1.9 to 8.6 mg per 100 ml. All had proteinuria and ketonuria. The cadmium reaction was negative in all and the thymol turbidity positive in one. A further 7 patients without jaundice had bilirubin and urobilin present in their urines. All patients recovered. Of Herold's 25 patients 8 had a serum bilirubin of more than 1 mg per 100 ml, with 2 peak values of 4.4 and 6.7 mg per 100 ml. Bilirubinuria was present in those with a serum bilirubin of more than 1.5 mg per 100 ml. Direct reacting bilirubin was positive in 19 and the galactose tolerance test impaired in 16. Thorling reports 6 patients with hyperemesis and jaundice. Five had associated or preceding pruritus, which run parallel with the vomiting in three. Three patients had an elevated alkaline phosphatase. The thymol turbidity was normal in all. Both serum transaminases may be increased in the more severe cases: SGOT up to 82 units, SGPT up to 283 units (Durst and Strauss).

No liver biopsies have been performed in this disease. Sheehan reported in

1939 19 autopsy cases of patients dying from hyperemesis. Those with a duration of symptoms of more than 6 weeks were slightly jaundiced. Thirteen had cerebral symptoms prior to death which were interpreted as Wernicke's encephalopathy. Histologically the liver was normal in 7 and showed in 12 a slight fatty infiltration which was considered insignificant and did not lead to necrosis. A specific liver lesion has not been found and most reported histological changes could also be due to starvation and avitaminosis.

The incidence of hyperemesis gravidarum appears to be on the decline. Guttmacher reports that in 1937 one in every 150 pregnant patients had to be hospitalised for hyperemesis, while in 1957 the the figure was only 1 in 974. In reviews on jaundice during pregnancy no series since 1940 reports more than 6 patients with jaundice due to hyperemesis (see Table 4). The clinical problem encountered will be mainly one of differential diagnosis from the prodromal phase of viral hepatitis, which should not be too difficult when tests such as serum transaminases and thymol turbidity are employed.

Jaundice in hyperemesis may recur in successive pregnancies.

Jaundice in vomiting of late pregnancy
Apart from hyperemesis gravidarum which occurs in the first trimester and almost always clears spontaneously by the 12th week of gestation, there is a syndrome of "pernicious vomiting in late pregnancy" occurring usually between the 33rd and 37th week. Almost always an underlying cause like pyelonephritis, other infections or pre-eclampsia is found. Sheehan reports an autopsy series of 16 such cases, of which 4 had a serum bilirubin elevation to maximally 2 mg per 100 ml in the last few days of life. The livers showed histologically no significant changes or a slight fatty infiltration.

Clinically this syndrome never presents as a case of jaundice. The term should best be abandoned, because rarely does vomiting appear to be "idiopathic".

Jaundice in toxemia of pregnancy
Toxemia of pregnancy is accompanied by an increased incidence of abnormal so-called liver function tests, but liver function on the whole is not impaired. Among 44 patients Dieckmann et al. found in 51 % a positive cephalin flocculation and in 43 % a positive thymol turbidity test. A slight increase in bromsulfalein retention was noted by Christhilf and Bonsnes. Serum alkaline phosphatase was elevated in 75 % of Mukherjee's 100 toxemic patients, compared to a 28 % incidence in his normal pregnant controls. The observed range was 12.5 to 16.5 King—Armstrong units in mild and 13.4 to 29.5 units in severe cases. Alkaline phosphatase closely parallels the clinical course in eclampsia and increases with the number of convulsions. Serum glutamic oxalacetic transaminase and lactic dehydrogenase are often elevated in the more severe cases (Kubli). Within the first 36 hours after admission SGOT was elevated in all of Crisp et al.'s 64 patients, with values above 100 units (maximum 244 units) in all severe cases. A rapid fall in SGOT indicated a good prognosis.

Jaundice is rare in toxemia, occurs

late in the course and often suggests a grave prognosis. The bilirubin increase in 17 % of Dieckmann et al.'s 44 patients was only slight. Of Verhage's 96 patients with toxemia only 11 had icterus, 2 of which died. In Sheehan's autopsy series of 90 cases only 10 were jaundiced. Sheehan believes the icterus to be due to hemolysis, as his jaundiced patients had hemoglobinuria during life and hemoglobin casts in the kidney tubules at autopsy.

Histological liver lesions, so striking at autopsy, are absent in mild and even in some far advanced cases on liver biopsies (Ingerslev and Teilum III). Of 15 severe cases with convulsions only 5 showed definite liver lesions in Antia et al.'s biopsy series. In Sheehan's opinion histological changes occur only during the last two days of life.

The liver lesions reflect the basic vascular disorder. Characteristic findings consist of fibrin thrombi in the sinusoids of the periportal zone. Similar thrombi occur in other organs. In the liver they obstruct sinusoidal blood flow and cause sinusoidal dilatation, which leads to necrosis of clusters of hepatic cells (often wrongly called fibrinoid necrosis) and finally to hemorrhagic necrosis of the periportal zone. If the patient has been in shock centrolobular necrosis may be superimposed and the areas of hemorrhagic necrosis may become confluent and form large blood pools. An inflammatory reaction is characteristically absent. Liver lesions in eclampsia are therefore interpreted as a terminal event (Sheehan, Ingerslev and Teilum III, Dietel 1947, Dieckmann 1952, Antia et al. 1958).

The rare case of jaundice due to toxemia of pregnancy will hardly present clinically as an icterus of unknown origin.

5) Indications for interruption of pregnancy because of jaundice

Interruption of pregnancy because of a disease causing jaundice during pregnancy is never indicated with the possible exception of acute fatty metamorphosis of pregnancy.

This statement will not be questioned when applied to chronic idiopathic hyperbilirubinemias, or to drug-induced intrahepatic cholestasis and tetracycline toxicity. In the rare case of jaundice due to common duct obstruction surgery on the biliary tract can be performed during gestation. When jaundice of this kind develops after the 36th week surgery may be delayed until after delivery. Treatment in jaundice due to pyelonephritis with septicemia is directed at the infection.

Intrahepatic cholestasis of pregnancy is definitely not an indication to terminate pregnancy. Although an induced interruption of pregnancy will "cure" the disorder, such a cure will occur in all cases after spontaneous delivery. Symptoms are never so distressing as to justify a shortening of the jaundiced period, since pruritus can be effectively relieved by cholestyramine. Many interruptions have been performed, especially in the recurrent form, but usually by physicians who were not familiar with this disease and its absolute and constant benignity.

An interruption of pregnancy has

often been advocated in severe cases of viral hepatitis. As has already been pointed out in the respective chapter, no evidence exists that the course of viral hepatitis is affected by pregnancy itself. Pregnancy is influenced by viral hepatitis in a tendency to premature deliveries. However, spontaneous abortions in severe cases of hepatitis do not improve the course of the disease, and furthermore a turn to the worse has been observed after spontaneous abortions. In addition, any narcosis or surgery is very poorly tolerated in severe cases of hepatitis, which again is a strong point against a surgical termination of pregnancy.

The course of a patient with liver cirrhosis is generally not influenced by pregnancy. It has already been pointed out, that cirrhotic females with pregnancies present in a way a selection of cirrhotics with fairly good liver function, as in severe cases of cirrhosis fertilisation is rare. Pregnancy may possibly increase portal hypertension by an increase in intraabdominal pressure. In pregnant cirrhotics with hematemesis due to esophageal varices successful porto-caval shunts have been performed. The rare case in which liver function decompensates critically during pregnancy would probably have a poor prognostic outlook even without pregnancy. Furthermore, in such a case surgery is as poorly tolerated as in severe viral hepatitis. For all these reasons, an induced termination of pregnancy appears not indicated in cirrhosis.

In rare cases of severe hyperemesis gravidarum or severe toxemia of pregnancy a termination of gestation may become necessary. The indications for an interruption of pregnancy will be based on general obstetrical principles and will not be based on the presence or absence of jaundice. In hyperemesis gravidarum jaundice does not carry a grave prognosis. In toxemia of pregnancy jaundice occurs only in the severe cases and its presence may be an additional point for the obstetrician in favour of a termination of gestation. Valuable guides for the prognostic outlook in toxemia of pregnancy are the serum alkaline phosphatase and the serum transaminases.

Acute fatty metamorphosis of pregnancy is probably a valuable and furthermore the only indication to terminate pregnancy because of jaundice. In order to be successful a Caesarian section has to be performed very early in the course, which necessitates an early and correct diagnosis for which a liver biopsy is nearly indispensable. As performance, embedding and reading of a liver biopsy usually takes two days in the most favorable circumstances, it may be necessary to avoid this delay and to take a decision without a biopsy, based on the typical clinical symptoms and signs.

Interruption of pregnancy may be indicated in some hemoglobinopathies which are known to take a deleterious course under the influence of pregnancy (especially S—C, S—S and C—C disease) and in some hemolytic anemias during pregnancy not responding to medical treatment. In these instances the decision will be taken because of hemolysis and not because of jaundice. Jaundice, if present, is mild anyhow in these disorders.

III. Recurrent jaundice during pregnancy

Clear definitions of the different diseases disguised under the term "recurrent jaundice during pregnancy" are hampered by the similarity of the clinical course between many of these disorders, which are nearly all benign as evidenced by their recurrence during successive pregnancies. Puyo wrote in his thesis in 1953: "Les travaux publiés, malgré le nombre de cas rapportés et le nombre de données (clinique, biologique et histologique) souvent réuni, sont mal utilisable quand on désire se faire une idée des particularités de ces ictères." Furthermore, the majority of case reports are but sparsely documented with laboratory data and rarely verified by liver biopsies. The problem of delivering the pregnant patient usually takes precedence over the problem of investigating the cause of jaundice, especially as jaundice is mild in this syndrome and clears rapidly after delivery.

1) Historical note

Recurrent jaundice during pregnancy has to our knowledge first been noted by Hoffman in 1872 ("une jeune femme, laquelle à chaque grossesse devenait ictérique peu de temps avant d'accoucher"). The first case report giving some details was published by Ahlfeld in 1881. Up to 1910 15 cases were known in the medical literature. During the next 12 years only 1 case was published. Interest in this disease continued to be minor, with 11 cases reported between 1923 to 1935 and 5 cases reported from 1940 to 1948. The years 1950 to 1959 brought 30 new cases and the discovery of further patients promises to be profuse in the 1960's.

Many of the early authors concluded that in the case they described jaundice was in some way linked to the state of gestation. With the description of additional cases it became apparent that at least two thirds of all patients with recurrent jaundice during pregnancy had similar and typical symptoms (defined on page 36) and that they therefore must represent a definite disease entity. This disease, now called recurrent intrahepatic cholestasis of pregnancy, has been clearly and fully described by two Swedish authors, Svanborg in 1954 and Thorling in 1955. Both workers also defined the first attack, i.e. the non-recurrent form of the same disease. The intrahepatic cholestasis mechanism has, however, been definitely expressed in a case report by Perreau in 1953 and was probably first alluded to by Boreel in 1924 at Van den Bergh's department. The first liver biopsies in this disease were performed by Ljunggren in 1956 and Gros in 1958.

The difficulties in clearly separating the different disorders causing recurrent jaundice during pregnancy are best exemplified in the largest single series of cases (Perreau and Rouchy 1961): Of the 9 cases in the report only 7 conform to the diagnosis of recurrent intrahepatic cholestasis of pregnancy. Case II had histologically the features of cirrhosis of the liver and case III is an example of recurrent pruritus during pregnancy.

2) Recurrent intrahepatic cholestasis of pregnancy

Nomenclature

Recurrent jaundice of pregnancy has originally been used as a purely descriptive term, meaning the occurrence of jaundice during successive pregnancies. As more and more cases were described in the literature, the term assumed the meaning of a specific disease (Magnani 1924, Schwalm 1932, Perreau 1953). Finally, "recurrent jaundice of pregnancy" was used by Svanborg in 1954 to include also the non-recurrent form of the same disease (i.e. first attack in just one pregnancy). While most cases described under this heading are examples of intrahepatic cholestasis of pregnancy, other forms of jaundice during pregnancy may also present as recurrent jaundice during successive gestations (discussed under differential diagnosis of recurrent jaundice), which further confuses the issue. In Thorling's opinion, the term "recurrent jaundice of pregnancy" designating a form of jaundice peculiar to pregnancy, has become redundant.

We share Thorling's opinion and reject the term "recurrent jaundice *of* pregnancy" as meaning a specific disease, but we propose to retain the term "recurrent jaundice *during* pregnancy" as a purely descriptive one without etiological implications, just as the term "jaundice" alone is descriptive without implying a specific disease entity.

The disease formerly called "recurrent jaundice *of* pregnancy" is in our opinion best termed recurrent "intrahepatic cholestasis of pregnancy". A multitude of other names have been used for its designation. The term most frequently employed in the older literature is "icterus gravidarum" (Ahlfeld 1881, Becking 1896, Von den Velden 1904, Boreel 1924) or "Schwangerschaftsicterus" (Benedict 1902, Mayer 1906) and "Graviditätsicterus" (Brauer 1903). However, the same term served also to include all forms of jaundice during pregnancy. The word "idiopathic" was then added, as in "idiopathic hepatopathy of pregnancy" (Ljunggren 1956), "idiopathischer Schwangerschaftsikterus" (Eppinger 1937, Gros 1958, Wilken 1958) and "idiopathic jaundice of pregnancy" (McAllister and Waddell 1962, King and Kerrins 1963). The etiology of the disease is certainly unknown and the term "idiopathic" is at present justified, but "acute fatty metamorphosis of pregnancy" is also idiopathic and does also occur only in pregnant women (Moore 1963). "Benign jaundice of pregnancy" (Orellana et al. 1961) and "Hépatite bénigne de la grossesse" (Caroli et al.) appear correct, but not precise enough.

Attempts at a pathogenetic description are expressed in the next group of terms. "Hepatosis" (Sheehan 1961) or "obstetric hepatosis" (Ikonen 1964) ex-

TABLE 10. Recurrent jaundice during pregnancy. Classification of cases used in review of literature

Category	Description	Number of cases	Tables
I	Recurrent intrahepatic cholestasis of pregnancy with liver biopsies	23	Table 11
	I A) with laboratory data and details on clinical course 18		Tables 13, 16
	I B) without further details 5		Table 18
II	Probable recurrent intrahepatic cholestasis of pregnancy, with sufficient laboratory data, but without liver biopsies	20	Table 17
	II A) with details on clinical course 15		Table 14
	II B) without further details 5		Table 19
III	Recurrent jaundice during pregnancy with details on clinical course. No biopsies, no or scarce laboratory data	12	Table 15
IV	Recurrent jaundice during pregnancy, number of gestations mentioned only	26	Table 20
V	Recurrent jaundice during pregnancy, no details reported	23	Table 21
VI	Recurrent jaundice during pregnancy, sufficient details reported to exclude intrahepatic cholestasis of pregnancy (liver biopsy in 6 cases)	28	—
Total cases of recurrent jaundice during pregnancy		132	
VII	Non-recurrent jaundice during pregnancy, considered to represent possibly intrahepatic cholestasis by original author or by reviewer	267	Table 22
	VII A) cases with liver biopsy 33		Table 12

References are given in the respective tables.

cludes an infectious agent, but has been applied by others to jaundice seen in hyperemesis and eclampsia (Gros 1958). "Hépatite toxi-gravidique" (Caroli et al. 1954) might as well be used in eclampsia with jaundice and is therefore nonspecific. "Endogenous hepatotoxemia of pregnancy" (Thorling 1955) has the same disadvantage as "idiopathic" and could also include acute fatty metamorphosis of pregnancy. Furthermore the term calls for a counterpart, "exogenous hepatotoxemia of pregnancy", which was used by Thorling for jaundice during pyelonephritis in gestation, but which might also be employed in other septicemias, in chloroform poisoning, or in drug-induced jaundice.

In a designation for the disease the intrahepatic cholestasis mechanism was first alluded to by Caroli et al. (1954) in the term "forme dite choléstatique pure des hépatites ictérigènes de la grossesse", later changed to "ictère choléstatique de la grossesse" by Perreau and Rouchy (1961). "Intrahepatic cholestasis of pregnancy", finally, has been used by Haemmerli and Wyss for the presentation of their first 5 cases (Annual Meeting of the Swiss and German Gastro-

TABLE 11. Liver biopsies in recurrent intrahepatic cholestasis of pregnancy. (Category I)

Year	Author	Author's case number	Number of pregnancy	Time of biopsy (days)*	Duration of jaundice at biopsy (weeks)
1956	Ljunggren	?	1	early pp late pp	?
1958	Gros	1	8	2 pp	6
1959	Svanborg & Ohlsson	?	?	ap pp	? ?
1959	Dölle & Martini	11	4	p	5
1960	Pieragnoli et al.	1	2	5 pp	2
1961	Belvederi & Finotti	1	2	5 ap	4
		2	2	ap	4
1962	Cahill	1	2	?	3—4
		2	5	?	?
1962	Dietel	1	2	7 pp	3—4
1962	Hausheer & Lauer	1	4	1 pp	6
		1	5	10 pp	1
1963	Béraud et al.	1	2	pp	4
1963	King & Kerrins	1	3	5 pp	3
1963	Moore	1	6	4 pp	4
		2	3	early pp	?
		2	4	at p	11
1964	Ikonen	L.A.	2	6 pp	?
		S.V.	5	ap	<1
		A.S.	2	14 pp	?
		A.P.	5	21 pp	<1
1966	Haemmerli & Wyss	B	2	21 pp	3
		C	2	3 pp	1
		E	3	2 pp	2
		F	6	at p	2

* ap = before delivery,   pp = after delivery,   at p = on day of delivery.

enterological Associations, September 30th 1960, in Zürich) and was first employed as title in a report describing own cases by Orellana and Osorio in 1963. The term is also used in Sherlock's textbook.

Henceforward we will employ the terms "intrahepatic cholestasis of pregnancy" and "recurrent intrahepatic cholestasis of pregnancy" to designate a specific disease. The term "recurrent jaundice *during* pregnancy" will be used as a descriptive one for the classification of diseases of different etiology.

Findings	Needle biopsy	Surgical biopsy taken during:	Abdominal operations without liver biopsy
Marked cholestasis	+		
Minimal cholestasis	+		
Mild cholestasis	+	(Peritoneoscopy)	
Cholestasis, irregular and focal	+		
Normal	+		
Normal		Caesarian section	
Mild cholestasis	+		
Minimal cholestasis	+		
Centroacinar bile pigment in liver cells	+		
Cholestasis	+		
Cholestasis	+		
Cholestasis	+		
Minimal cholestasis	+		
Normal	+		
Focal cholestasis	+		Exploratory laparotomy T-drain in common duct
Cholestasis	+		
Normal	+		Interval cholecystectomy
Minimal cholestasis	+		
Minimal cholestasis		Caesarian section	
Cholestasis	+		
Normal		Abdominal hysterotomy	
Normal	+		Caesarian section
Normal		Abdominal hysterectomy	
Centroacinar bile pigment in liver cells		Exploratory laparatomy	Surgical sterilisation
Minimal cholestasis	+		
Mild cholestasis	+		
Minimal cholestasis		Abdominal hysterotomy	

Material for review of world literature
Whenever an attempt is made to delineate a newly emerging disease entity by reviewing all published case reports in the literature, it appears wise to include in such a review only cases in which the diagnosis is beyond doubt. In intrahepatic cholestasis of pregnancy no parameter singly or in combination with others is specific and none will provide an unquestionably correct diagnosis. However, two features will allow to restrict any errors in diagnosis to an acceptable minimum:

1. recurrence of the same syndrome (defined on page 36) during successive pregnancies.
2. a liver biopsy compatible with intrahepatic cholestasis.

These two criteria are met in 14 reports covering a total of 23 patients. In only 18 of these sufficient information is available on clinical course and laboratory data. These 18 patients underwent a total of 70 pregnancies, 4 of which terminated in an early abortion, 9 were uncomplicated, 11 were associated with pruritus only and 47 showed the full syndrome with pruritus and jaundice. These 47 pregnancies will form the basis for our review.

A combined total of 132 cases of recurrent jaundice during pregnancy has been published in the literature. For the purpose of this review the cases have been divided into 6 categories according to their documentation (see Table 10). Occasionally it has become necessary to allot different cases contained in a single report into different categories.

Category I will be used to discuss liver biopsy findings, categories I A and II to discuss laboratory data. Categories I A and II A will serve for the description of the clinical course. The 61 cases in categories III, IV and V provide insufficient data for a critical evaluation. The 28 cases in category VI do definitely not belong to the disorder called intrahepatic cholestasis of pregnancy and will be discussed under the section on differential diagnosis.

The 267 patients with the non-recurrent form of (possible) intrahepatic cholestasis of pregnancy (category VII) are added to complete the review. They will be discussed but briefly to point out some discrepancies with the confirmed cases or to point out some possible diagnostic pitfalls.

The reports covering category I and II cases originate from Sweden, Finland, England, Ireland, Germany, Switzerland, France, Italy, Poland, Canada, the United States of America and Chile. Additional countries contributing to category III—V cases are Holland, Austria, Roumania and Argentina and a category VII case is reported from Belgium.

Liver biopsies

In 25 pregnancies of 23 patients a total of 27 liver biopsies have been performed (category I, see Table 11). Of the 27 biopsies 20 were blind percutaneous needle biopsies, 1 consists of a needle biopsy taken during peritoneoscopy and 6 are surgical biopsies (Seydl's case with a normal biopsy 2 months after the disappearance of jaundice has been put into category II).

The findings are rather uniform. The liver architecture is intact. There is no liver cell damage. Neighbouring liver cells look alike. Minor deviations from the normal, consistent with those usually seen in uncomplicated pregnancy occur as an expression of an increased regenerative activity. They consist of Kupffer cell proliferation and mobilization, mild thickening of the framework, PAS positive granules in the Kupffer cells, some PAS containing macrophages in the portal spaces and of incipient ballooning of liver cells in the centroacinar areas.

TABLE 12. Liver biopsies in non-recurrent intrahepatic cholestasis of pregnancy. (Category VII A)

Year	Author	Total cases	Histological diagnosis	
			Cholestasis	Normal
1947	Nixon et al. (case 14)	1	1	—
1953	Puyo (case 4)	1	1	—
1956	Ljunggren	6	5	1
1959	Svanborg & Ohlsson	4	3	1
1961	Katz et al.	4	3	1
1961	Van Woert & Kirsner	1	—	1
1963	Brown et al.	3	3	—.
1963	Myhre	1	—	1
1963	Orellana & Osorio	8	7	1
1964	Ikonen	2	1	1
1964	Gros	2	2	—
1966	Haemmerli & Wyss (unpublished)	2	2	—
	Combined	35	28	7

The only truly abnormal finding is confined to the centroacinar area. Some bile canaliculi contain bile plugs. The canaliculi are of normal caliber or occasionally slightly dilated. The liver cells surrounding the centroacinar bile canaliculi contain bile pigment and may show an accumulation of fine basophilic granules. The portal tracts are not involved.

The histological picture is consistent with the diagnosis of intrahepatic cholestasis. In only one case (Ljunggren) is cholestasis described as marked. In 15 others bile stasis is mild or even minimal. In 2 instances only biliary pigment in the centroacinar liver cells and no capillary bile plugs were found. In 5 cases liver biopsy was described as normal. Three authors have stressed the fact, that cholestasis, if present, is irregular and focal (Svanborg and Ohlsson, Bé-

raud et al., Haemmerli and Wyss). On different sections from the same biopsy bile plugs may be present in one slide and absent in the other (Haemmerli and Wyss). If cholestasis is not carefully looked for, it may be missed, as often only a few bile thrombi are seen on one slide and bile pigment deposition in the liver cells is not impressive. This may explain 3 normal readings, the biopsies of which were taken before delivery in 1, during delivery in 1 and 4 days after delivery in a third case. The 2 other normal readings occurred in biopsies taken 14 and 21 days after delivery, where cholestasis may well have disappeared.

In 2 cases 2 biopsies were taken during the same pregnancy (Ljunggren, Svanborg and Ohlsson). The cholestasis had regressed in both instances during the second biopsy, taken after delivery. In another case with a biopsy taken 3 weeks after delivery biliary pigment was found in the centroacinar liver cells, but bile canaliculi were normal. Apart from this rapid improvement after delivery, no correlation appears to exist between intensity of histological cholestasis and intensity of jaundice, duration of icterus before biopsy or time relation of biopsy to date of delivery.

It is remarkable how little impressive histological cholestasis in this disease is when compared with the clear-cut clinical and biochemical "obstructive pattern", especially considering the often violent pruritus of the patients.

A further 35 biopsies have been performed in the non-recurrent form of intrahepatic cholestasis of pregnancy (category VII A, see Table 12). The histological findings were identical, with 28 biopsies showing cholestasis and 7 read as normal. The 3 cases of so-called "hepatitis" during pregnancy with normal liver biopsies reported by Ingerslev and Teilum in 1951 may represent 3 further examples.

The 3 non-recurrent cases biopsied by Brown et al. were examined by electron microscopy. The microvilli of the bile capillaries were swollen and occupied most of the lumen. Within the liver cells dilatation and vacuolization of the profiles of the endoplasmic reticulum was seen, with occasional complete desintegration of ergastoplasm. No controls in uncomplicated pregnancy were done and no recurrent case of intrahepatic cholestasis of pregnancy has yet been examined by electron microscopy. Furthermore, two of the three cases were clinically atypical: case 1 had splenomegaly and case 2 no pruritus and a prodromal phase of malaise, weakness and anorexia. For these reasons, the findings of Brown et al. cannot yet be accepted as representative for recurrent intrahepatic cholestasis of pregnancy.

Biopsies have been performed in 6 other instances of recurrent jaundice during pregnancy (Nixon et al. cases 16 and 19, Perreau and Rouchy, case II, Caroli et al. case 3, Lebon et al., Justin—Besançon et al.). The histological findings differed from those described above, but so did the clinical and biochemical findings. These cases do not represent intrahepatic cholestasis of pregnancy and will be discussed under the section on differential diagnosis.

Gross anatomical findings and radiological gallbladder examinations
No woman died of the disorder and no post-mortem examinations have been performed.

Ten of the 23 patients in category I underwent 11 surgical abdominal interventions, in 7 of which liver biopsies were taken (see Table 11). The interventions consisted of 3 surgical interruptions of gestation in the 3rd or 4th month because of jaundice (Ikonen cases S. V. and A. P., Haemmerli and Wyss, case F), 2 exploratory laparatomies because of jaundice (Béraud et al., Haemmerli and Wyss, case B), 1 peritoneoscopy because of jaundice (Gros), 3 Caesarian sections (Moore case 2, Dölle and Martini, Ikonen case A. S.), 1 surgical sterilisation on the day of spontaneous delivery (Haemmerli and Wyss case B) and 1 cholecystectomy in the interval between 2 pregnancies, with normal biliary system at operation (Moore case 1).

The liver was considered to be of normal appearance in 10 instances and to be slightly enlarged in 1 patient (Ikonen, case A. P.). The spleen was found to be normal in all cases. During peritoneoscopy Gros described the liver as being of normal size, shape and consistency, its surface as smooth, glistening, of grey-brown colour with a greenish tint. A close-up view revealed a fine greenish stippling.

One case in category I had gallstones (Haemmerli and Wyss, case F). They were discovered after the 6th pregnancy. No cholecystectomy was done. This woman had only a single, questionable episode of biliary colic 11 years previously and none during the next 16 years. Three further patients of categories II—V had gallstones. The patient of Katz et al. (category II B) underwent a cholecystectomy for cholelithiasis after her 3rd pregnancy. Her first pregnancy was asymptomatic, her 2nd to 5th complicated by pruritus only and her 6th to 8th were associated with pruritus and jaundice. Case O. S. of Ikonen (category IV) was cholecystectomized for gallstones after her 2nd pregnancy and was jaundiced again in her 3rd gestation. Another patient with gallstones is Cahill's case 4 (category V, no details).

In Moore's case 2 (category I A) the gallbladder was removed after her 6th pregnancy despite of a normal preoperative cholecystogram and despite of normal findings at operation. Interestingly enough, her next pregnancy was asymptomatic. Her first 3 pregnancies were, however, asymptomatic too. Non-

icteric pregnancies following icteric ones have been observed in 3 instances without cholecystectomy and without evidence of gallbladder disease (King and Kerrins, Ikonen case A. S., Haemmerli and Wyss, case C).

These several observations make a causal relationship between gallstones and jaundice, or between cholecystectomy and absence of jaundice unlikely.

Radiological gallbladder examinations were performed in 8 of the surgically explored cases and in an additional 6 patients without surgical procedures in category I. Of the latter normal results were obtained in all (Cahill case 1, Pieragnoli et al., King and Kerrins, Hausheer and Lauer, Ikonen case L. A., Haemmerli and Wyss, case C). Of the patients with normal cholecystography after delivery three had a previous radiological examination during the height of jaundice, all showing nonfilling of the gallbladder (Béraud et al., Hausheer and Lauer, Haemmerli and Wyss, case C). In category II A cholecystograms were performed in 3 cases with normal results (Jodkowski and Chojecka, McAllister and Waddell, Simmons).

A very interesting observation was made in the case of Béraud et al. In this woman jaundice set in in the second month of gestation and lasted until after delivery at term. At 4 1/2 months of gestation an exploratory laparatomy was performed. Despite normal macroscopic findings and a normal operative cholangiogram a T-drain was inserted into the common duct. Bile flow from this tube was normal in volume, colour and viscosity, and the intensity of jaun-

51

TABLE 13. Clinical course in recurrent intrahepatic cholestasis of pregnancy. Cases verified by liver biopsy (category I A)

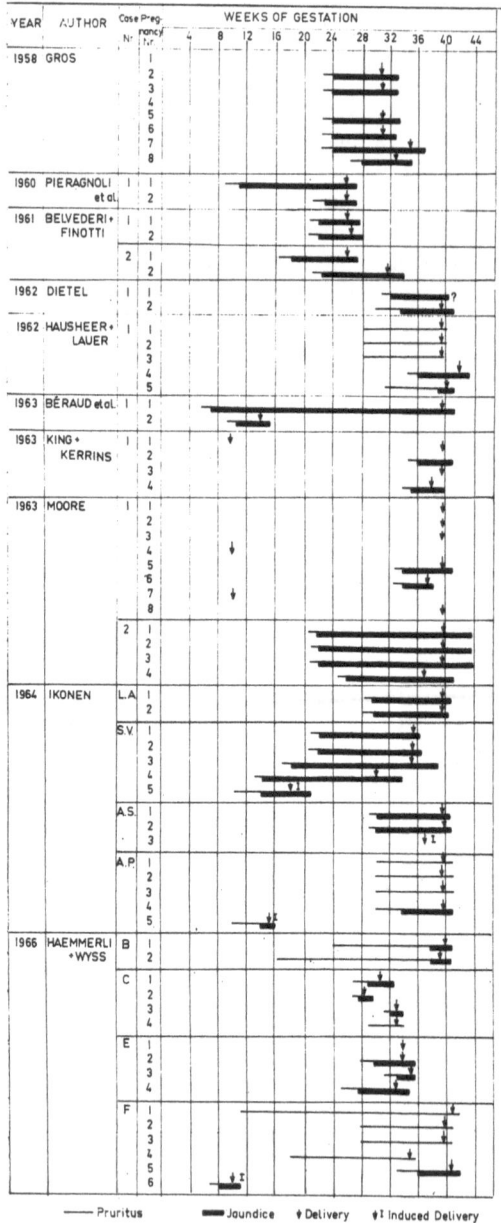

TABLE 14. Clinical course in recurrent intrahepatic cholestasis of pregnancy. Cases without liver biopsy, but with adequate laboratory data (category II A)

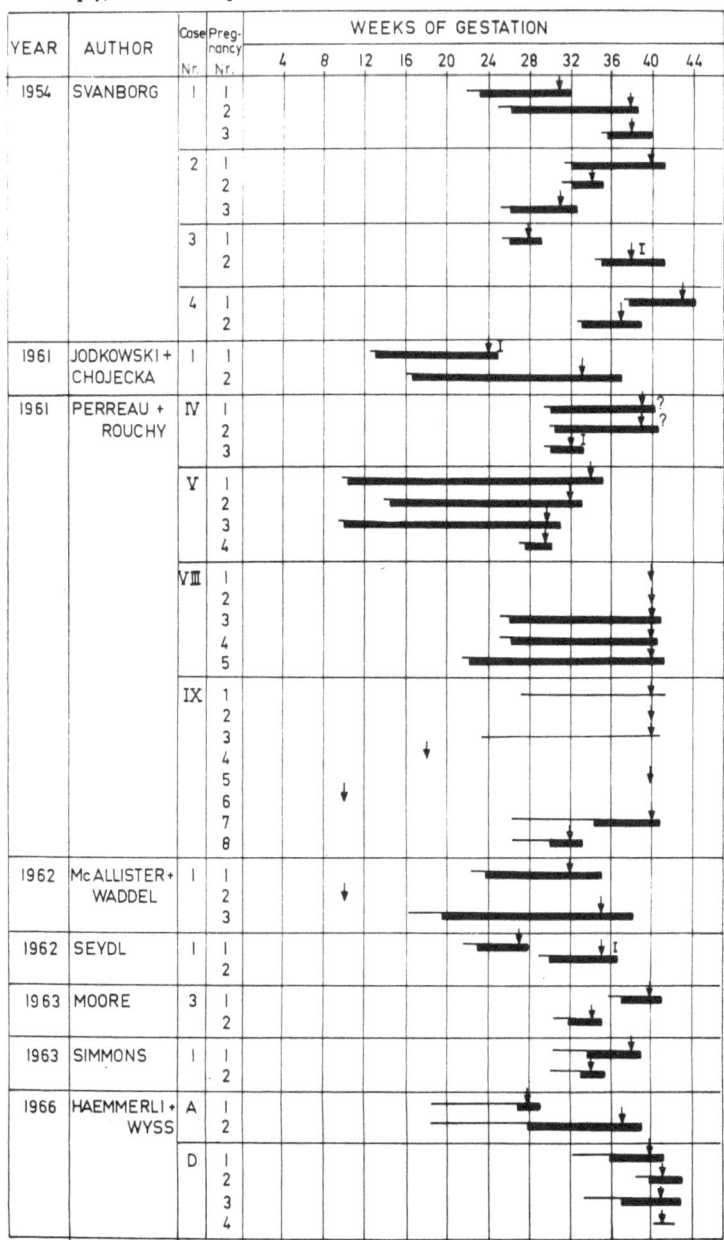

TABLE 15. Clinical course in pruritic recurrent jaundice during pregnancy. Cases without adequate laboratory data. Possibly examples of recurrent intrahepatic cholestasis of pregnancy (category III)

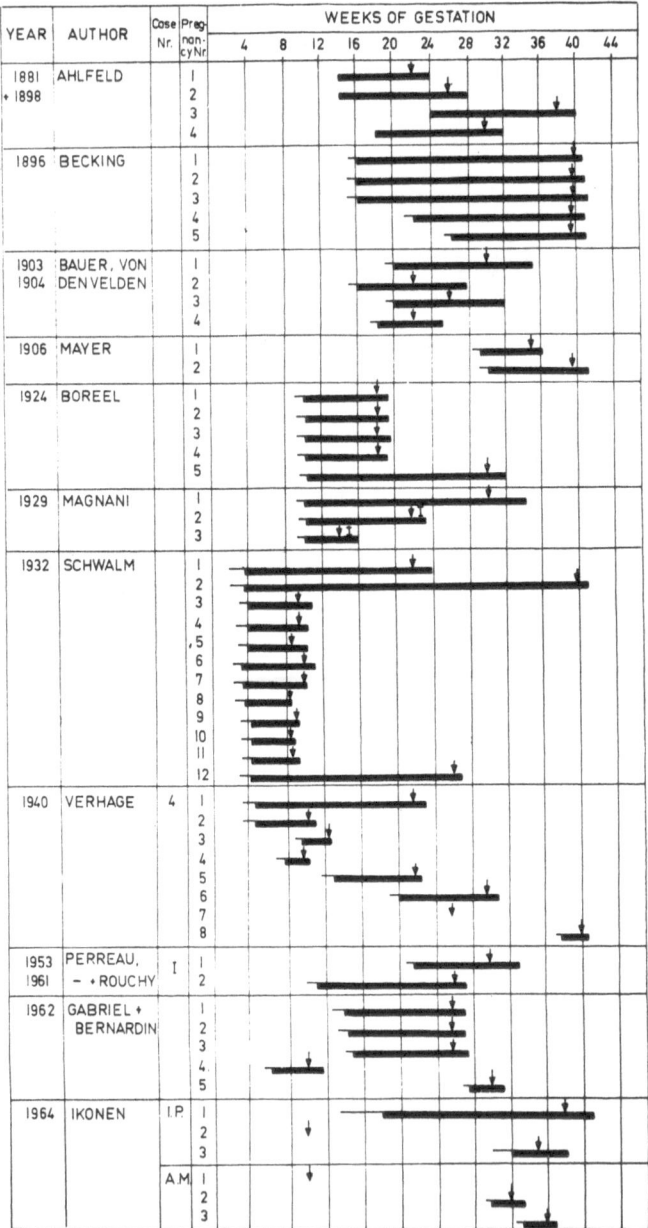

dice did not change during the long drainage period.

Symptoms and signs

The disease has been observed in all age groups during the childbearing period. The clinical course in categories I A, II A and III is graphically summarized in Tables 13, 14 and 15 respectively.

Pruritus is the first symptom to occur and dominates the clinical picture throughout the whole course in this disorder. Pruritus is usually violent and involves the trunk or the extremities or both. Most authors note that the palmar and plantar surfaces of hands and feet may be involved. When pruritus lasts for more than two weeks excoriations (scratch marks) usually appear on the skin. In a rare case they may become secondarily infected and result in an impetigonous rash (Haemmerli and Wyss, first pregnancy of case F). Pruritus usually leads to insomnia which renders the women tired and irritable. Pruritus precedes jaundice usually by 1—2 weeks, but may begin up to 22 weeks earlier (Haemmerli and Wyss, second pregnancy of case B).

In some instances pruritus is the only clinical symptom of liver dysfunction and jaundice does not occur at all. In these cases pruritus may be of long duration (up to 30 weeks, in first pregnancy of case F, by Haemmerli and Wyss). Pruritus gravidarum without jaundice appears to be a "forme fruste" of intrahepatic cholestasis of pregnancy.

Intrahepatic cholestasis of pregnancy has been called "jaundice of late pregnancy" and it has been stated that jaundice always begins during the last 4 months of gestation (Svanberg and Ohlsson). This applies to the majority of the cases but there are many exceptions. Mean and median onset of jaundice among 47 icteric pregnancies in category I A is in the 26th week of gestation or just before the beginning of the last trimester. The observed range of onset varies between the 7th and the 39th week of gestation, with 2 pregnancies in the 7—8th week, 2 in the 11th, 3 in the 14th, 2 in the 18th, 14 in the 22nd to 24th, 1 in the 26th, 9 in the 28th to 30th, 7 in the 32nd to 34th, 4 in the 35th to 36th and 3 pregnancies in the 38th to 39th week of gestation.

In 7 cases of category I A jaundice was noted between the 7th and 14th week of gestation. In addition, jaundice began in the third month of gestation during the second to fifth pregnancy in Cahill's case 2 (category I B). Of 37 icteric pregnancies in category II A onset of jaundice was in 5 between the 10th and 16th week, in 5 between the 20th and 24th week, in 8 between the 26th and 28th week, in 8 between the 30th and 32nd week, in 7 between the 33rd and 36th week and in 4 between the 37th and 40th week. Category III includes possibly other forms of jaundice besides intrahepatic cholestasis of pregnancy. Still, it may be of interest to note that icterus began in all 12 pregnancies of Schwalm's case in the first month of gestation. Onset of jaundice in the 3rd month occurred in 5 pregnancies of Boreel's and in 3 pregnancies of Magnani's case.

Of course, statistical figures dating onset of jaundice are in a way fallacious.

The patient herself will notice her jaundice often well after its true onset. On the other hand serum bilirubin elevation was noted very early before onset of clinical jaundice in at least 3 instances with onset of jaundice in the first trimester. These patients were carefully followed by their physicians because of the history of their previous pregnancies with jaundice (Ikonen cases S. V. and A. P., Haemmerli and Wyss, case F).

Duration of jaundice from its observed onset until spontaneous delivery varied in 42 instances of category I A between 1 and 33 weeks, with a mean of 8.1 and a median of 6 weeks. Duration of 1 to 2 weeks occurred in 7 instances, of 3 to 4 weeks in 7, of 5 to 6 weeks in 8, of 7 to 8 weeks in 6, of 10 to 11 weeks in 4, of 12 to 13 weeks in 4, of 15 to 18 weeks in 5 and of 33 weeks in 1 instance.

In category II A duration of jaundice from its observed onset until spontaneous delivery varied in 33 instances between 1 and 24 weeks, with a mean of 7.7 and a median of 5 weeks. Duration of 1 to 2 weeks occurred in 9 instances, of 3 to 4 weeks in 6, of 5 weeks in 3, of 8 to 9 weeks in 6, of 12 to 16 weeks in 5 and of 17 to 24 weeks in 4 instances.

During jaundice or just preceding its onset the urine is described as dark by all patients. The stool colour is light in some instances, definitely normal in others, and not noticed by the patient or physician in most cases.

The general health of the patients is not impaired during the jaundiced stage. They feel well — apart from the irritation and lack of sleep resulting from itching — and continue without difficulties their daily work, including heavy manual labor (farmer's wife). This is in marked contrast to the reduced general condition in viral hepatitis. In intrahepatic cholestasis of pregnancy there are no prodromal or general symptoms such as fever, nausea, vomiting, liver pains, arthralgias, anorexia — again in contrast to the clinical picture in viral hepatitis.

The 3 cases reported in the two Italian papers are the only ones to have associated symptoms apart from pruritus and jaundice. The first symptom during the first pregnancy in all 3 cases was severe pain in the right upper quadrant of the abdomen, radiating to the right shoulder in two cases. In the patient of Pieragnoli et al. and in case 1 of Belvederi and Finotti this was associated with fever up to 38° centigrade. These symptoms are probably not related to intrahepatic cholestasis of pregnancy and did not recur in the two cases during the second icteric pregnancy. Case 2 of Belvederi and Finotti had some pains in the right upper abdominal quadrant during two pregnancies. A cholecystogram was normal in the case of Pieragnoli et al. The 2 cases of Belvederi and Finotti had the same gastrointestinal symptoms already before their first pregnancy.

No woman in categories I and II presented evidence of toxemia of pregnancy. Toxemia and pyelitis were noted in Ikonen's case O. S. (category IV).

Physical examination is unrevealing except for the presence of jaundice and scratch marks. The liver is rarely and the spleen never palpable. As examination of these patients is usually performed near term palpatory findings may be difficult to elicit. On the other hand, liver and spleen size were normal in all 10 cases with surgical abdominal explorations. Easy bruising or echymosis would be exspected in cases with prolonged prothrombin time (usually occurring in cases with jaundice of long duration), but has never actually been observed in these patients.

In no case of categories I and II did onset of jaundice precede onset of pruritus and in no case did jaundice disappear before delivery. After delivery, whether spontaneous or induced, jaundice decreases rapidly and disappears usually within 1—2 weeks. In 46 instances in category I A jaundice disappeared within 1 week in 18, within 2 weeks in 21, within 3 weeks in 1 and within 4 weeks in 6 instances. The 6 instances with prolonged post-delivery jaundice are confined to 2 patients: Moore's case 2 and Ikonen's case S. V. Moore's case 2 forms an exception in another respect: the intensity of jaundice increased during the first postpartum week. The same phenomenon occurred once in a case of category II A (Jodkowski and Chojecka, second pregnancy). Jaundice lasted for 6 weeks after delivery in 3 pregnancies of the non-verified case of Brauer and Von den Velden (category III).

Pruritus disappears before jaundice subsides. The only dissenting opinion is that of Svanborg and Ohlsson. All other authors agree that pruritus may disappear completely on the first postpartum day in some cases and decreases markedly in intensity immediately after delivery in all other instances, to disappear completely before jaundice vanishes.

There is no evidence that intrahepatic cholestasis of pregnancy leaves any residual liver damage, but long-term and careful follow-up examinations have been few in number. Slightly elevated alkaline phospatase levels have been observed 4 months and 1 year after an icteric pregnancy in 2 cases (Haemmerli and Wyss, cases B and F), but repeat examinations later on were normal. In one case bromsulfalein retention was 24 % in 45 minutes 2 months after delivery (Béraud et al.) and in another 7 % 1 year after delivery (Ikonen, case S. V.). Long-term follow-up examinations of 1 to 5 years with normal results were obtained in 10 cases (Thorling cases 39 and 56, Svanborg and Ohlsson 3 cases, Cahill case 1, Haemmerli and Wyss, cases A, B, D, and F). Pavel's case 1 (category IV) developed probable hepatitis 3 months after the last of 6 gestations with jaundice, but recovered rapidly and was well at the age of 65 years.

Laboratory data

Laboratory data of patients in category I A and category II A are summarized in Tables 16 and 17 respectively. The values given are the most abnormal ones recorded in the individual pregnancy for each single test. The several test results given for a single individual were not necessarily obtained on the same day. For example, peak bilirubin levels were usually observed before delivery, but peak alkaline phosphatase levels a few days after delivery. Furthermore, few patients have been serially examined and the "maximal" abnormal tests summarized in the tables may well be submaximal,

TABLE 16. Recurrent intrahepatic cholestasis of pregnancy
Cases with detailed laboratory data and liver biopsy (Category I A)

Year	Author	Number of case and pregnancy	Urine			Serum Bilirubin mg/100 ml		Alkaline phosphatase Bodansky units	Cholesterol mg/100 ml
			Bilirubin	Urobilin	Urobilinogen	Total	Direct		
1958	Gros	1—8	+		↑	4.6	2.9	N	221
1960	Pieragnoli et al.	1—2	+	+		6.8	5.0		400
1961	Belvederi & Finotti	1—2	+	+		6.8	5.0		400
		2—2	+	+		5.3	4.0		386
1961	Dietel	1—2	+	—		3.5		13⁺	280
1962	Hausheer & Lauer	1—4				4.5	1.9	22*	314
		1—5				3.2	1.3	15*	
1963	Béraud et al.	1—1	+			5.5	4.1		213
		1—2	+			5.6	4.2	28	240
1963	King & Kerrins	1—2				3.5	2.2		
		1—4				3.7	3.0	6.8	
1963	Moore	1—6				2.1		28	
		2—4				3.5		26	
1964	Ikonen	L.A.—2	+			2.8			
		S.V.—5				1.2		7	255
		A.S.—2				1.5			515
		A.S.—3				0.5		4	400
		A.P.—4	+			3.5		6.8	
		A.P.—5	—			1.2		4.2	
1966	Haemmerli & Wyss	B—1	(+)	—	N	3.5		11.6	287
		B—2	—	—	N	3.6		21.2	590
		C—1	+	+	N	5.9		17.5	290
		C—2	+	—	↑	3.6		14.6	450
		C—3	+	+	↑	3.6		14.4	420
		E—2	+	—	N	4.2		11.4	
		E—3	+	—	N	4.5		13.4	360
		E—4	(+)	—	N	4.5		11.8	300
		F—5	(+)	(+)	N	5.0		12.6	333
		F—6	↑	—	↑	3.1		12.7	200

N=normal   ↑=increased   +=positive   —=negative   * Conversion from Bessey-Lowry units

because examinations have not been performed during the peak abnormality.

Serum bilirubin determinations have been obtained in 29 pregnancies of the 18 patients in category I A. Jaundice is always of mild degree. The maximal recorded value was 6.8 mg per 100 ml. This value is surpassed three times in category II A with 7.8 (Haemmerli and Wyss, case A), 8.0 (Perreau and Rouchy

| Transaminases Wróblewski units | | Prothrombin time % | Thymol turbidity MacLagan units | Zinc sulfate flocc. Kunkel units | Cephalin-cholest. flocculation | Takata reaction | Serum iron γ/100 ml | Bromsulfalein retention % | Galactose tolerance test |
SGOT	SGPT								
			2				68		
25	53				—			↑	↑
25	53		N		--			↑	↑
		42	N					↑	
↑↑	↑↑	100				+	109		
34		100	5.7		(+)				
50			N		0				
		100	7					22	
		70	2		0			25	N
920		89	1		0				
			3						
			2						
			N						
200			1						
107	230	33					110		
75	100								
95									
76	160							18	
30	22	60			0	N	50−205		N
69	50		2.2	3.2	0	N	50−100	10	N
79	53	70			0	N	45−130		
52	53	100	4.9	7.9	0	N	115−180		
238	175	50	4.5	4.7	0		130		
90	90	85			0	N	20−190		
106	145				0	N	40−140		
142	220		3.5		0	N	90−155		
183	226	30			0	N	130−250	13	N
150	197	82	4.4	6.4	0	N	355		

+ Conversion from King-Armstrong units.

case VI) and 8.4 mg per 100 ml (McAllister and Waddell). The direct-reacting serum bilirubin fraction, determined in 10 instances of category I A, is responsible for most of the total serum bilirubin elevation. Bilirubinuria was found in 17 of 20 instances. Bilirubinuria may be short-lasting or intermittent, and can therefore easily be missed (Thorling, Haemmerli and Wyss). Urobilinogen is

TABLE 17. Recurrent intrahepatic cholestasis of pregnancy
Cases with detailed laboratory data, but no liver biopsy (Category II)

Year	Author	Number of case and pregnancy	Urine Bilirubin	Urine Urobilin	Urine Urobilinogen	Serum Bilirubin mg/100ml Total	Direct	Alkaline phosphatase Bodansky units	Cholesterol mg/100 ml
1954	Svanborg	1−2				3.8		10+	
		1−3				2.6		7+	
		2−1				3.5		28+	
		2−3				5.1		16+	
		3−2				2.6		10+	
		4−2				1.6		8+	
1955	Thorling	39−3				2.1		6+	
		51−2				3.0		14+	
		56−1				2.3		14+	
1961	Jodkowski & Chojecka				N	6.5		11.8	235
1961	Katz et al.					3.6	1.4	15	334
1961	Perreau & Rouchy	IV—3	+			2.6			342
		V—4	+			4.0			460
		VI—2	+			8.0			170
		VIII—5	+			2.5		9*	388
		IX—8	+			6.8			240
1962	McAllister & Waddell		+			8.4	3.0	6.6*	
1962	Seydl					3.1		15	
1963	Moore	3−1				2.6	1.9	8*	
		3−2				3.9		16*	
1963	Simmons	1−1				2.5		15*	
		1−2	+			3.0		19*	
1966	Haemmerli & Wyss	A—2				7.8		6	231
		D—1	(+)	+	↑	3.6		20.7	213
		D—2	−	+	↑	2.4			384
		D—3	−	−	N	1.3		22.0	370
		D—4	−	−	↑	0.8		19.4	350

N=normal   ↑=increased   +=positive   —=negative   * Conversion from King-Armstrong units

present in normal or increased amounts, but is never completely absent from the urine. Urobilin was found in 6 of 14 instances.

Consistent with the clinical and histological feature of cholestasis there is as a rule an elevation of alkaline phosphatase and cholesterol. One or the other or even both these tests may be normal, however, in an occasional case.

Alkaline phosphatase, determined in 22 pregnancies of 14 patients in category I A was normal in 2 pregnancies, between 4 and 7 Bodansky units in 4

SGOT	SGPT	Prothrombin time %	Thymol turbidity MacLagan units	Zinc sulfate flocc. Kunkel units	Cephalin-cholest. flocculation	Takata reaction	Serum iron γ/100 ml	Bromsulfalein retention %	Galactose tolerance test
			5			N			
			2			N			
			1						
			1			N			
			3			N			
			1			N			
		115	1			+			
		89	N	N	0				
		96	3						
		↑				+			
52	94	100	N			N		16	
		100							
		77							
80	48		8		2+			16	
	↑	80			0				
			1						
			2						
			3						
			N	2					
			2	2					
						N			N
		37			+	N	45 − 160		
91	77				+	N	55 − 160	23	N
66	78	100	3	5.1	(+)	N	100 − 160	23	
28	27				0	N	100 − 200		

+ Conversion from Buch-Buch units.

pregnancies and between 11 and 28 Bo-dansky units in 16 gestations. The find-ings in category II A correspond in general to the ones in category I A. As most figures given for category II A had to be converted into Bodansky units from other units, no data will be tabu-lated. Serum cholesterol, determined in 13 pregnancies of category I A, was be-low 250 mg per 100 ml in 3 and between 255 and 590 mg per 100 ml in 10 gesta-tions. In 12 pregnancies of category II A serum cholesterol varied between 170 and 460 mg per 100 ml.

The elevation of serum cholesterol is seldom more pronounced than that seen in uncomplicated pregnancies (Ikonen), whereas serum alkaline phosphatase elevation is — when present — usually much more marked than the usual elevation observed towards term in uncomplicated gestations (Thorling). There is no correlation in the single case between elevation of serum bilirubin, alkaline phosphatase or cholesterol.

Serum electrophoresis, performed in 15 pregnancies of 5 patients reported by Haemmerli and Wyss, fits also into the pattern of biochemical cholestasis. There is a decrease in serum albumin, a slight increase of alpha-1 and a moderate increase of alpha-2-globulins, a usually pronounced increase in beta-globulins and normal or slightly decreased gamma globulins. In every case the beta-globulin fraction is higher than the gamma-globulin fraction. The electrophoretic changes represent an exaggeration of those seen in uncomplicated pregnancy. Total proteins are somewhat decreased as in normal gestation.

The serum turbidity and flocculation tests are normal as a rule, with few, but only borderline exceptions (Perreau and Rouchy, case VIII).

Prothrombin time is normal or only slightly prolonged in the majority of cases. It may be prolonged to critical levels whenever jaundice is of long duration. This is the only test that shows such a correlation. Of 17 pregnancies in category I A prothrombin time was below 60 % in 7 instances, 3 of which being around 30 %. Prolongation of prothrombin time is entirely due to a deficiency in the Vitamin K dependent coagulation factors II, VII and X (Haemmerli and Wyss) and is readily corrected by the application of Vitamin K.

Serum glutamic oxalacetic transaminase may be normal or increased. In 21 pregnancies of 12 patients in category I A it was normal in 4, between 50 and 100 units in 9, between 100 and 240 units in 7 patients and 920 units in the case reported by King and Kerrins. Serum glutamic pyruvic transaminase, determined in 14 pregnancies of 7 patients, was normal in 1, between 50 and 100 units in 6 and between 100 and 230 units in 7 gestations. It was not determined in the case with the exceptionally high SGOT. Besides the high SGOT found in the case of King and Kerrins, 2 other recurrent cases of Ikonen (not specified which ones) had similar high levels: SGOT 716 and SGPT 875 in one case and SGOT 450 and SGPT 565 in the other. SGPT was higher than SGOT in 9 of 16 cases with both determinations (category I A and Ikonen's cases). Five cases in category II with determination of the transaminases show mild to moderate elevations.

The 3 cases with very high transaminases are astonishing. As they fit in all other regards into the general picture of intrahepatic cholestasis of pregnancy, and as one of these cases has been biopsied, they are tentatively accepted in this review. For practical diagnostic purposes, however, it appears wise for the present to regard a level of 250 units as the upper limit usually seen in this disease.

Serum 1-phospho-fructaldolase was elevated to 8.4 units and serum sorbit dehydrogenase up to 7.6 units in case E of Haemmerli and Wyss. In serial determinations during two pregnancies of this patient both enzymes paralleled the behaviour of the serum transaminases closely.

Bromsulfalein retention is always increased during jaundice. The recorded values in 8 cases of category I A and 4 cases in category II varied between 10 % and 25 % after 45 minutes. A special modification using a single intravenous injection of 800 mg bromsulfalein was employed in the three Italian cases of category I A. This test revealed a decreased hepatic uptake of bromsulfalein and an increased cholestatic index in all.

In contrast to the increased bromsulfalein retention, urinary galactose excretion after a 40 g oral loading dose is always normal. (4 tests in category I A and 2 in II A, in 4 of 6 tests simultaneous bromsulfalein test).

There is no evidence of hemolysis in this disorder. No erythrocyte survival studies have been performed and a mild hemolysis as a contributary phenomenon is therefore not excluded. Hemoglobin is usually normal for pregnancy. The lowest recorded hemoglobin levels are 63 % (Hausheer and Lauer), 66 % (Haemmerli and Wyss, second pregnancy of case B) and 67 % (Jodkowski and Chojecka). Reticulocyte counts are not increased. Urobilinogenuria cannot be used as a criterium for hemolysis in the presence of disturbed liver function. Serum iron levels behave erratically (Ikonen, Haemmerli and Wyss), with both abnormally low and abnormally high levels (up to 355 microgm per 100 ml) in the same pregnancy. Nearly all increased levels were found before delivery, decreased levels both before and after. There is no correlation between serum iron and hemoglobin. There is also no correlation between serum iron and serum transaminases such as occurs in viral hepatitis (Haemmerli and Wyss).

Total leucocyte and differential counts are normal or show a leucocytosis and/or shift to the left as in uncomplicated pregnancies. Non-protein nitrogen is never elevated.

Laboratory data before and after delivery

Long and serial pre-delivery laboratory examinations have been performed only in the 6 cases reported by Haemmerli and Wyss. These periods were of 14, 15, 22, 24, 62 and 125 days duration. It is probable but not conclusively proved, that an elevation of the serum transaminases first indicates the onset of the full syndrome. However, bilirubin elevation lags but a few days behind. Serial observations in cases with a long preicteric pruritic phase are necessary to settle this question. Serum alkaline phosphatase and serum cholesterol are usually elevated before the serum bilirubin or the transaminases. The significance of this elevation is difficult to evaluate as both these parameters are increased in the last trimester of most normal pregnancies.

In cases with jaundice of short duration serum bilirubin usually increases towards delivery. In cases with jaundice of long duration serum bilirubin rapidly reaches a plateau. It may remain steady or fluctuate and even decrease slightly

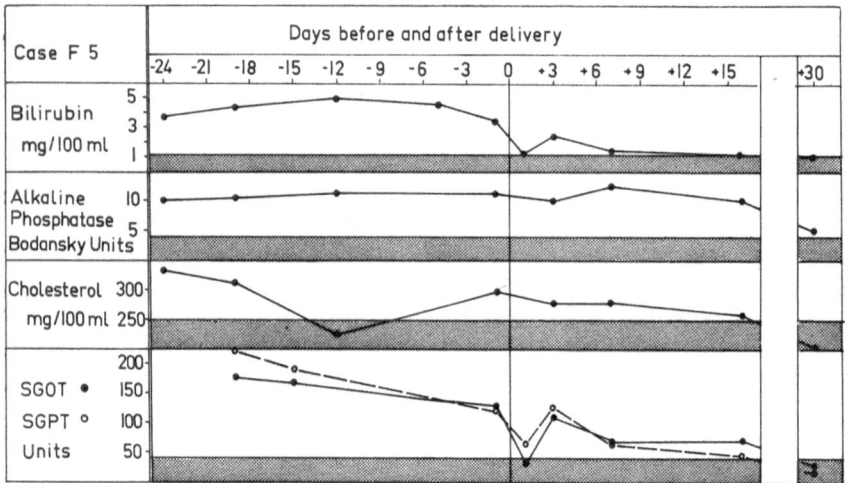

Fig. 1. Example of laboratory data in recurrent intrahepatic cholestasis of pregnancy. (case F, fifth pregnancy, Haemmerli and Wyss 1966).

toward delivery (Haemmerli and Wyss, case A).

After delivery serum bilirubin and serum transaminases begin to decrease immediately and are, together with urinary bile pigments, the first tests to become normal again. Serum alkaline phosphatase may continue to increase for 4 to 10 days after delivery (Haemmerly and Wyss) and is the last test to become normal. Mild elevations may persist for up to 2 months after delivery.

A curious phenomenon was observed by Haemmerli and Wyss in 2 cases. Immediately after delivery there was a transient "dip" or return to normal of serum bilirubin and serum transaminases, only to reach pre-delivery levels again within 24 hours. A gradual improvement occurred thereafter (see Fig. 1). It it not clear whether this phenomenon is a rule or an exception. Because of its short-lasting transient nature it will easily be missed if serial laboratory determinations in 8 to 10 hour intervals are not performed during the first day after delivery.

Obstetrical course, incidence of premature deliveries and child survival

No obstetrical complications occurred during delivery in category I A. There is a single mild complication in category II A: patient D reported by Haemmerli and Wyss had a blood loss of 750 ml during her first delivery. Her prothrombin time was 37 % of normal. The child's prothrombin time was 0 % and it died despite immediate Vitamin K therapy from massive intracranial hemorrhage. The bleeding in the mother stopped spontaneously and did not necessitate blood transfusions.

The incidence of premature deliveries is high in the combined series. Among

TABLE 18. Recurrent intrahepatic cholestasis of pregnancy
  Cases with liver biopsies, but no details on clinical course (category I B)

YEAR	AUTHOR	CASE NR	PREGNANCIES
1956	LJUNGGREN		▤ ▤
1959	SVANBORG+OHLSSON		▤ ▤
1959	DÖLLE +MARTINI		▤ ▤ ▤ ▤
1962	CAHILL	1	▤ ▤
		2	□ ▤ ▤ ▤ ▤

TABLE 19. Recurrent intrahepatic cholestasis of pregnancy
  Cases with laboratory data, but no details on clinical course (category II B)

YEAR	AUTHOR	CASE NR	PREGNANCIES
1955	THORLING	39	□ □ ▤ ▤
		51	▤ ▤
		56	▤ ▤
1961	KATZ et al.		□ ▤ ▤ ▤ ▤ ▤ ▤ ▤
1961	PERREAU +ROUCHY	VI	▤ ▤ ▤

Legend for Tables 18 and 19 see Table 20.

43 pregnancies with jaundice and spontaneous delivery in the 18 cases of category I A there were 23 premature deliveries and 20 deliveries at or near term. However, this kind of statistics is treacherous in a way, because 22 premature deliveries occurred in 7 women, and 19 deliveries at term in 10 women. In these cases every delivery of the single individual was either at term or premature (see Table 13). In just one case is a premature delivery combined with a delivery at term (Béraud et al.).

These general conclusions are also evident in category II A. Premature delivery correlates neither with time of onset of jaundice in relation to stage of pregnancy nor with the intensity or the duration of jaundice. Furthermore premature delivery appears to be independent of intrahepatic cholestasis of pregnancy itself. Case E of Haemmerli and Wyss delivered prematurely in 4 pregnancies, the first of which was uncomplicated. Similarly, case C of Haemmerli and Wyss delivered prematurely

TABLE 20. Recurrent jaundice during pregnancy
Cases reported with few details (category IV)

YEAR	AUTHOR	CASE NR	PREGNANCIES
1902	MÜLLERHEIM		□ ◧ ◧
1910	NASON		□ □ A ◧ ◧ ◧ ◧ ◧ □ □ □
1910	ROLLESTON		■ ■ ■ ■
1924	BOREEL	mother of case	◧ ◧ ◧ ◧ ◧ ◧ ◧
1935	PEL		◧ ◧ □ ◧ ◧
1953	PUYO	2	■ ■ ■
1954	DOWIE		◧ ◧
1955	MEYER	1	◧ ◧
		2	◧ ◧
1957	PAVEL et al.	1	■ ■ ■ ■ ■ ■
		2	■ ■ ■ A◧ ■ ◧
1958	WILKEN	2	◧ ◧
1959	SVANBORG + OHLSSON		■ ■ ■
			■ ■
			■ ■
		sister	■ ■
1961	PERREAU + ROUCHY	VII	◧ A ◧
		sister of case VI	■ ■ ■ ■ ■ ■
1961	ORELLANA et al.		■ ■
			■ ■ ■
1961	SHEEHAN		■ ■ ■
1963	ORELLANA + OSORIO		■ ■ ■ ■
			□ □ ◧ ◧ ■ ■ ■
1964	IKONEN	O.S.	■ ■
		L.V.	■ ■
		M.S.	□ ■ ■

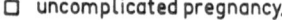

□ uncomplicated pregnancy,

◧ pregnancy with pruritus

■ pregnancy with pruritus and jaundice

◧ pregnancy with jaundice, pruritus not mentioned, not negated.

A abortion

66

in 4 pregnancies, the last of which was complicated by pruritus without jaundice.

Thus, premature delivery appears to be a feature of the single individual. The overall high incidence remains still to be explained. Perhaps whatever mechanism causes intrahepatic cholestasis of pregnancy may independently also cause premature delivery, with no direct causal relationship between jaundice and premature delivery.

Of 23 children born prematurely 10 died shortly after birth. Of the 20 children born after the 36th week 6 died during delivery mainly from intrauterine asphyxia. The already mentioned death of an infant with a prothrombin time of 0 % from intracranial bleeding and a similar incident in a non-recurrent case of Thorling's are probably unrelated to the jaundiced mother's coagulation deficiency, because extremely low prothrombin times are encountered not infrequently in newborns from healthy mothers.

No baby was jaundiced in categories I and II. Several jaundiced babies were observed in 3 non-verified cases of category IV (Nason, Rolleston, Pavel et al. case 1). Erythroblastosis foetalis is not excluded in these cases, 2 of which were reported in 1910. There were 2 congenital malformations in category III, both occurring in the same mother (case I. P., Ikonen): the first child died with ileal atresia 6 weeks after birth and the second was stillborn with a ventricular septal defect. Jaundice began during the 5th month in the first and during the 8th month in the second gestation, so that a causal relationship to the malformations is very unlikely.

TABLE 21. Recurrent jaundice during pregnancy. Cases without any details reported (Category V)

Year	Author	No of cases
1872	Hoffman	1
1905	Kehrer	4
1923	Eppinger	1
1927	Holmer	1
1957	Wewalka	3
1961	Meeroff	1
1962	Cahill (cases 3 and 4)	2
1962	Friedberg	4
1963	Orellana and Osorio	2
1964	Ikonen	4
	Total	23

Clinical course of successive pregnancies in the individual patient

The pregnancies of categories I A, II A and III are summarized in Tables 13, 14 and 15 respectively, the pregnancies of categories I B, II B and IV in Tables 18, 19 and 20. Category V cases without details are mentioned in Table 21.

A glance at Tables 13 and 14 will rapidly show, that the clinical course in this disease is by no means uniform. About the only existing rule is that jaundice occurs some time before delivery and disappears rapidly thereafter, whether delivery is spontaneous or induced.

It has been stated by Svanborg and Ohlsson that the disease runs a similar course in the individual patient in repeated pregnancies. This generalization is true only to a certain extent and is even contradicted by the 4 cases reported by Svanborg in detail 5 years earlier (category II A). An apparent similarity exists in the course of 8 of 18 cases in category I A. However, among these 8 cases only the one of Belvederi and Finotti is reported with exact details of all pregnancies. In the other 7 reports (Gros, Dietel, Hausheer and Lauer, 4 cases of Ikonen) the descriptions of all except the last pregnancy of the cases are lumped together (for example: "Jaundice usually appeared in the 24th week and lasted until 2 weeks after delivery"), and therefore we assume that the "similarity of the course" is more fictitious than real. If a history on previous pregnancies is obtained during the last pregnancy only, not to much weight should be put upon a woman's recollection. Wherever detailed charts for each pregnancy were available for retrospective review (as in the series of Haemmerli and Wyss) similarity is less striking.

Jaundice does not necessarily occur during every pregnancy of the single individual. Jaundice in every pregnancy was present in only 9 of 18 cases in category I A. Seven of these 9 cases underwent 2 pregnancies only and may therefore not be representative for the full spectrum of possibilities in this disease.

Jaundice when present is not necessarily of the same intensity during successive pregnancies. Jaundice of equal intensity was noticed in the same 9 of 18 cases mentioned above: 7 patients with 2 pregnancies, 1 with 4 (Moore, case 2) and one with 5 pregnancies (Ikonen, case S. V.).

The other 9 patients in category I A

show a varying symtomatology during successive gestations. It may be significant, that all these cases underwent 3 or more gestations (mean 5.2, maximum 8).

In the patient reported by King and Kerrins only the second and the fourth pregnancy were associated with pruritus and jaundice, whereas the first and third were uncomplicated. In case 1 of Moore only 2 of 6 fullterm pregnancies were symptomatic, the first three and the last one being uncomplicated.

In 5 cases the syndrome appears to progress in intensity during successive pregnancies. In 3 patients the first 3 or 4 pregnancies were complicated by pruritus only, the following two showing the full syndrome with jaundice (Hausheer and Lauer, Ikonen case A. P., Haemmerli and Wyss case F). In the other 2 cases the first pregnancy was asymptomatic, with the full syndrome in the following gestations (Gros, Haemmerli and Wyss case E). In addition, Cahill's case 2 (category I B) conforms to this pattern, but no details are given.

In 2 cases a definite improvement is noted in successive pregnancies with the last one being completely asymptomatic (case A. S. by Ikonen, case C by Haemmerli and Wyss).

Among the 15 cases in category II A (Table 12) jaundice was about equal in successive pregnancies in 12 patients, 8 of which with 2, 3 with 3 and 1 with 4 pregnancies. A progression in intensity is shown in the cases VIII and IX by Perreau and Rouchy, with the first several pregnancies asymptomatic or pruritic only. An instructive example of decreasing intensity is provided by case D of Haemmerli and Wyss, with peak serum bilirubin levels of 3.6, 2.4, 1.3 and 0.8 mg per 100 ml in 4 successive pregnancies.

In category V there are 2 remarkable cases. In the patient of Dowie the interval between the first and second pregnancy with jaundice was 12 years. The case of Nason had jaundice only in the 4th to 8th of her 11 pregnancies. In the 7th and 8th pregnancy jaundice disappeared about 10 days before delivery, so that the possibility of diagnosis other than intrahepatic cholestasis of pregnancy exists.

No definite statement as to the frequency of recurrence in successive pregnancies can be made because non-recurrent cases have been excluded from this survey. Thorling reported 10 multiparas with gestation after an icteric pregnancy. Three had again pruritus and jaundice, two pruritus only and 5 were asymptomatic during the next pregnancy.

Treatment

Intrahepatic cholestasis of pregnancy is a benign disorder with full recovery after delivery. One hesitates even to call it "liver disease". From the standpoint of therapeutic consequences it might as well be regarded as just a disordered function of little importance. Neither bed rest nor a dietary regimen are necessary and the "patient" may continue her normal daily life. Whenever jaundice is of longer duration (more than 2 weeks) the prothrombin time should be checked regularly. If this is not practicable Vitamin K can be given prophylactically.

Pruritus, the most annoying symptom, does not respond to antihistaminics

(Gros, Haemmerli and Wyss). Itching is easily abolished with cholestyramine, an ion exchange bile acid sequestrant, in the dose of 10 gm per day. When the drug is stopped pruritus recurs within 1 to 2 days. (Haemmerli and Wyss). Cholestyramine was also successfully employed in the non-recurrent case 3 of Brown et al. and in a case of pruritus gravidarum with slightly elevated alkaline phosphatase, cholesterol and transaminases but no jaundice (Haemmerli and Wyss, unpublished observation).

Intrahepatic cholestasis of pregnancy is definitely not an indication for an induced termination of pregnancy. An induced termination of pregnancy may lead to the loss of the child. It will certainly "cure" the mother's jaundice, but this will be cured anyhow after spontaneous delivery. As pruritus can now be easily controlled with cholestyramine there is no symptom which could demand a shortening of the jaundiced period. Today induced terminations of pregnancy are usually performed by physicians who are not familiar with the disorder and mistake it for a serious liver disease.

Antecedent or underlying hepato-biliary or gastrointestinal disease

The past history of patients with intrahepatic cholestasis of pregnancy is usually non-revealing except for the usual childhood diseases. Case B of Haemmerli and Wyss (category I A) had probable viral hepatitis at the age of 8 years. Nonspecific upper gastrointestinal disturbances before the first pregnancies were noted for 1 and 9 years respectively in the 2 cases of Belvederi and Finotti.

These symptoms recurred during their pregnancies (category I A). Ulcerative colitis of about 1 year's duration was diagnosed in the middle of the 12 year interval between the 2 pregnancies with jaundice of Dowie's case (category IV).

The 4 patients with cholelithiasis have already been mentioned in the paragraph on radiological gallbladder examinations.

Familial occurrence of intrahepatic cholestasis of pregnancy

Some patients with recurrent intrahepatic cholestasis of pregnancy have close relatives with a history of recurrent jaundice during pregnancy. None of these relatives has been examined in detail.

Jaundice during pregnancy occurred in 2 sisters of one of Cahill's cases (category I B or V, not stated which case). Case VI of Perreau and Rouchy (category II A) had a sister with jaundice during 6 successive pregnancies, each leading to premature delivery. Pruritus and jaundice were observed during one of several pregnancies in the mother of the case reported by both Brauer and by von den Velden (category III). The mother of Boreel's case (category III) was jaundiced during 7 pregnancies and the patient was the only surviving child, all others dying from prematurity. Two pregnancies with jaundice occurred in the older sister of a patient reported by Svanborg and Ohlsson (category IV).

The mother of case S. V. reported by Ikonen (category I A) had pruritus without jaundice during the 4th, 5th, 10th and 11th of her 13 pregnancies.

Pruritus with jaundice occurred once in a maternal cousin of the same case.

The two sisters with recurrent jaundice during pregnancy reported by both Benedict and Lovrich probably represent another disorder as both had hepatomegaly and one a marked splenomegaly in addition. An older sister and the mother of these two cases had uncomplicated gestations.

In Mayer's case (category III) the mother died from liver carcinoma and the father and one sister suffered from "chronic liver disease".

An inherited predisposition to intrahepatic cholestasis of pregnancy can neither be accepted nor be excluded from these observations.

Non-recurrent intrahepatic cholestasis of pregnancy

A total of 267 cases with a possible diagnosis of non-recurrent intrahepatic cholestasis of pregnancy have been published in the literature. The laboratory data are summarized in Table 22. In 35 cases liver biopsies were performed (see Table 12). Associated cholelithiasis, thought to be unrelated to jaundice, was found in 17 of 267 patients.

Many of these cases are incompletely documented and many may belong to quite different diagnostic categories. In 15 patients jaundice was associated with severe pyelonephritis (Van Woert and Kirsner, Laurijssens and Demeulenaere, Comerford, case 4, Thorling case 42, Ikonen 11 cases) and in 3 cases jaundice was associated with pyelitis and hemolysis (Thorling cases 40, 41 and 43). Toxemia of pregnancy was present in case 10 of Comerford and in 27 of Ikonen's cases. Two cases of Thorling had marked hypertension (number 64 and 67). Ten patients of Ikonen had anemia. Nine cases had no pruritus (Thorling 3 cases, Svanborg and Ohlsson 5 cases, Brown et al. case 2). Six cases listed are definitely not examples of intrahepatic cholestasis of pregnancy. In 4 of Thorling's cases jaundice disappeared well before delivery. Myhre's case had no pruritus, severe hypertension, marked hepatomegaly, an elevated serum amylase and a normal liver biopsy. Brown et al.'s case 1 had splenomegaly.

On the other hand, 8 cases published as viral hepatitis in the original reports have been included in Table 22 on the basis of their clinical and biochemical data (Nixon et al. case 14, Barry and O'Dwyer case 1, Comerford cases 1, 3, 5, 6, 7 and 9).

In Thorling's excellent monography on 72 patients with jaundice during pregnancy he writes: "Purely on the basis of the clinical signs and symptoms in the individual cases, the diagnosis of viral hepatitis appears to be possible in practically all the patients". He selected from this group 35 cases on two criteria: jaundice appeared in late pregnancy and the thymol turbidity test was negative. While the majority of this group may truly represent intrahepatic cholestasis of pregnancy, many will not. Wewalka pointed out that the thymol turbidity test may not be reliable during pregnancy. In his series thymol turbidity was positive in 82 % of patients with hepatitis outside of pregnancy, but in only 53.5 % of 58 cases with serum hepatitis (treatment for syphilis) during pregnancy.

The data in Table 22 are given for what they are worth. Just a few details will be pointed out.

It is remarkable that Orellana and Osorio collected their 59 cases within 2 years in a single hospital. Serum bilirubin levels are below 6.8 mg per 100 ml in all cases with one exception (case 2 of Brown et al. without pruritus, 8.7 mg per 100 ml). Alkaline phosphatase, cholesterol, prothrombin time, turbidity and flocculation reactions correspond to those in verified cases of recurrent intrahepatic cholestasis of pregnancy. The one high bromsulfalein retention of 50 % is from Brown et al.'s case 1 with splenomegaly. The biopsied case 2 of Gros had a 39 % retention, whereas all other bromsulfalein retention tests performed are between 14 and 28 % as in the verified cases. It will be remembered that in the verified category I A and II A cases the serum transaminases were below 250 units with three exceptions (King and Kerrins, Ikonen 2 cases). High values were also found in the non-recurrent case 3 of Brown et al. (SGOT 670, SGPT 220).

It must be concluded from this brief survey that the non-recurrent form of intrahepatic cholestasis of pregnancy is extremely difficult to diagnose with absolute certainty. The disease can easily be simulated by viral hepatitis with a benign course occurring late in pregnansy or by drug-induced intrahepatic cholestasis except that both these diseases have typical prodromal symptoms. For a diagnosis of non-recurrent intrahepatic cholestasis of pregnancy an absence of "hepatitis-like" prodromi and the rigid clinical, biochemical and histo-

TABLE 22. Non-recurrent intrahepatic cholestasis of pregnancy (267 cases) Diagnosis mostly not verified (Category VII)

Year	Author	Number of cases	Number of biopsies	Number of cholecystograms		Urine bilirubin	Serum bilirubin mg/100 ml	
				Total	Stones		Total	Direct
1947	Nixon et al. (case 14)	1	1				3.5	1.4
1953	Puyo (cases 4 &6)	2	1			+	1.6 − 5.0	
1954	Svanborg	3		2	2		2.1 − 5.1	
1955	Barry & O'Dwyer	1					2.0	
1955	Thorling	35		17	2		<5.8	
1956	Ljunggren	51	6	34	5		<6.5	
1959	Svanborg & Ohlsson	18	4	18	4		2.0 − 6.0	
1961	Katz et al.	7	4				<5.4	<3.0
1961	Orellana et al.	12					2.2 − 6.8	0.5 − 2.4
1961	Van Woert & Kirsner	1	1			+	2.2	1.5
1962	Comerford	6					1.6 − 5.0	
1962	Laurijssens & Demeulenaere	1					4.6	
1963	Brown et al.	3	3				2.2 − 8.7	1.3 − 2.8
1963	Moore	6						
1963	Müller & Felsch	20						
1963	Myhre	1	1	1			3.5	2.1
1963	Orellana & Osorio	59	8	21		+	1.3 − 6.8	0.3 − 3.1
1964	Ikonen	35	2	35	4	+	1.0 − 5.0	↑
1964	Gros	2	2	1		+	2.0 − 3.5	
1966	Haemmerli & Wyss (unpublished)	3	2			+	2.4 − 5.8	

N=normal   ↑=increased   +=positive   ° Conversion from Buch-Buch units   + Conversion from

logical criteria emerging from the review of the verified recurrent cases (category I A) must de demanded.

Pruritus is the prominent and probably compulsory symptom, but the presence of itching alone does not make the diagnosis of intrahepatic cholestasis of pregnancy. Pruritus appears to occur more frequently in all liver diseases during pregnancy than in liver disease outside of pregnancy. Thorling found pruritus in 17 of 23 cases of viral hepatitis during pregnancy (74 %) and believes that the pregnant state in some way favours the manifestation of this symptom in the presence of hepatitis. Martini et al. observed itching in 12 of 57 cases of hepatitis during pregnancy. Pruritus occurs also in hyperemesis gravidarum with jaundice and may be present in this disease without jaundice (Thorling). In two cases of acute fatty

Alkaline phosphatase Bodansky units	Cholesterol mg/100 ml	Transaminases Wróblewski units		Prothrombin time %	Thymol turbidity	Different flocculation tests	Bromsulfalein retention %
		SGOT	SGPT				
	630				N	N	
8−30°					N	N	
14				↑	N		
6−28°				3 ↑	N	N	
<20°				4:50−70	N		
				8 <50			
<26°				7 ↑	N	N	
<16+	<310	<76	<148	>55	N	N	14−24
12−36	215−331			83−100	N	N	
15	250			100	N	N	
6−21+					N		
15*		40	25		N		
13−14+	<279	55−670	62−220	N	N		28−50
		30−260	17−297				
11+		112	80	N	N	N	
9−36	29>300			13↑	N	N	
5−20*		2>300	2>300	20−100	4 ↑		
5−8		26−68	57−75	100	N	N	39
11−18	270−330	45−246	39−340	N	N	N	

King-Armstrong units   * Conversion from Bessey-Lowrey units.

metamorphosis of pregnancy marked pruritus was noted (Ober and Lecompte case 1, CPS case). Itching was also a feature in the two cases of jaundice with hemoglobinuria during pregnancy (Schaeffer, Meinhold).

Pruritus gravidarum

Itching has been defined as "an unpleasant cutaneous sensation which provokes the desire to scratch" (Thorling) or as "one of the seemingly mild symptoms which seems humorous to observers, but which may be desperately serious to the patient" (Kasdon). Itching is the most frequent cutaneous disturbance during pregnancy and occurs in a generalized or localized form, the latter as abdominal, vulvar or anal pruritus. Both forms usually occur during the second half of gestation.

Abdominal pruritus has been noted by Kasdon in 7 % of 42 women in the first trimester, in 20.9 % of 110 women during the second trimester and in 18.3 % of 213 women during the third trimester. The etiology is unknown.

The term pruritus gravidarum should be reserved for the generalized form. No statistics exist as to its frequency, but the syndrome is well known to all obstetricians. Circumstantial evidence favors the concept that pruritus gravidarum is a "forme fruste" of intrahepatic cholestasis of pregnancy. First of all, many cases of recurrent intrahepatic cholestasis of pregnancy will present with recurrent pruritus without jaundice during their first few gestations. Well documented examples have been published by Katz et al., Perreau and Rouchy case IX, Hausheer and Lauer, Orellana and Osorio, Ikonen case A. P. and Haemmerli and Wyss case F. Secondly in all cases of intrahepatic cholestasis of pregnancy jaundice is preceded and accompanied by pruritus. Thirdly, pruritus gravidarum has its onset in the second or third trimester and disappears with or shortly after delivery, i.e. its clinical course in relation to stage of gestation is the same as the course of intrahepatic cholestasis of pregnancy. Lastly, cases of pruritus gravidarum show some disturbed liver functions, which lie between those observed as "physiological" derangements during normal pregnancy and those seen in intrahepatic cholestasis of pregnancy.

Arfwedson 1953 and 1956 compared 100 pregnancies with pruritus gravidarum to 100 without. Serum bilirubin in those with pruritus was between 1 and 2 mg per 100 ml in 42 % and above 2 mg per 100 ml in 23 %, compared to only 6 % of determinations greater than 1 mg per 100 ml in normal pregnancy. Pathological bile components were found in 51 % of those with pruritus gravidarum and in 5 % of normal pregnancies. In 1956 Arfwedson and von Studnitz examined 42 women with pruritus gravidarum and 46 without during the last trimester. In those with pruritus there was a significant increase in total serum lipids, serum cholesterol, phospholipids and beta-lipoproteins, whereas alpha-lipoproteins were decreased. On serum electrophoresis there was a decrease in albumin and an increase in alpha-2 and beta-2 globulins in those with pruritus. Borglin found a SGOT elevation to 93 units in 1 out of 7 cases. Serum ornithyl carbamyl transferase was increased in 24 of 30 patients with pruritus (80 %), compared to only 15 % pathological results in normal pregnancies (Reichard et al.).

Few detailed case studies have been performed. In Thorling's 3 cases (number A, B and C) the serum bilirubin, thymol turbidity and cephalin flocculation were normal, and the alkaline phosphatase was increased up to 35 Buch and Buch units. Laboratory data in the 2 cases reported by Topp and Charles were: urine bilirubin positive, serum bilirubin 1.5 mg per 100 ml, alkaline phosphatase 35 King—Armstrong units and bromsulfalein retention 30 % in 35 minutes in case 1; urine bilirubin positive, serum bilirubin 1.0 mg per 100 ml, alkaline phosphatase 62 King—Armstrong units, cholesterol 295 mg per 100 ml, bromsulfalein retention 35 % at 35 minutes, transaminases, prothrombin time and flocculation tests normal in case 2. In an unpublished observation of Haemmerli and Wyss (wife of the second author) the following laboratory data were obtained: no abnormal urine bile components, total bilirubin 0,9 mg per 100 ml, direct-reacting bilirubin 0.3 mg per 100 ml, alkaline phosphatase 11.2 Bodansky units, serum cholesterol 330 mg per 100 ml, SGOT 69 units, SGPT 63 units, 1-phosphofructaldolase 4.5 units (normal up to 2.8 units), normal results for prothrombin time, serum iron and thymol turbidity.

Therapeutically, testosteron effectively controls itching but increases serum bilirubin levels (Arfwedson and von Studnitz). In the case of Haemmerli and Wyss cholestyramine in moderate dosis (6 gm per day) brought complete relieve, but itching recurred upon each attempted cessation of the drug. Cholestyramine was also successfully used in a case reported by Brown et al.

Pruritus gravidarum, once it occurs, has a marked tendency to recur in successive pregnancies (Thorling, Topp and Charles case 2) and may lead to intrahepatic cholestasis of pregnancy in a later gestation (Bjerregaard, Perreau and Rouchy case III).

3) Differential diagnosis of recurrent intrahepatic jaundice during pregnancy

The 28 cases in category VI are all examples of recurrent jaundice during pregnancy in which intrahepatic cholestasis of pregnancy can be excluded with near certainty on the basis of the published data. It is likely that some cases in categories III, IV and V would also have to be classified under a different heading if more data were provided for a critical evaluation of the orignal reports.

In 15 of the 28 cases the author's original diagnosis has been accepted in this review. In 8 cases a tentative reclassification was made (Perreau and Rouchy case II, Puyo cases Le B. and B. S., Nixon et al. case 16, Tylecote, Lantuéjoul and Chambraud, Ezès and Bourdon, Lebon et al.) and 5 cases could not be classified at all (Benedict, Lovrich, Vignes, Boquien et al., Justin—Besançon et al.). Sometimes our reclassification will appear arbitrary and occasionally different opinions as to the etiology of a particular case may be possible, even where a liver biopsy has been performed. For these reasons the case reports are recorded in some detail in this chapter.

Recurrent jaundice during pregnancy due to recurrent viral hepatitis or due to exacerbation of chronic anicteric hepatitis

Until recent years most French authors were convinced that recurrent jaundice during pregnancy is in all instances caused by viral hepatitis (Caroli et al.). In no case such an etiology is proved. In three cases, in which liver biopsies were performed, it may be possible.

The patient of Albano and Albano contracted viral hepatitis during her first pregnancy. After typical prodromal symptoms she developed jaundice in the 7th month, with a large tender liver, serum bilirubin up to 27.6 mg per 100

75

ml (direct reacting bilirubin 20.7 mg per 100 ml), both serum transaminases up to 1,100 units, positive zinc sulfate and thymol turbidity tests, normal alkaline phosphatase and bilirubinuria. She delivered several weeks later and was discharged with mild subicterus 2 weeks after delivery. In the interval she had some dyspeptic symptoms but no jaundice. Seven months later she was pregnant again. During the first month fever, dyspepsia, liver pains and subicterus set in. In the 5th month the serum bilirubin was 1.9 and the direct reacting bilirubin 1.0 mg per 100 ml. The urine was positive for bilirubin and urobilinogen, and there was an increase in gamma-globulins on electrophoresis. Alkaline phosphatase, the transaminases and all flocculation and turbidity reactions were normal. By the 7th month bilirubin had risen to 10.3 mg per 100 ml, SGOT to 300 units, SGPT to 400 units and the flocculation reactions were now positive. Liver biopsy showed an intact lobular architecture and massive round cell infiltration of the periportal spaces. On bed rest and medical treatment including steroids she improved, delivered at term and has since been anicteric.

It is possible that jaundice during the second pregnancy in this case is due to either a true recurrence of the initial viral hepatitis, dormant after the first pregnancy, or that it represents a clinical manifestation of an anicteric chronic hepatitis under the stress of pregnancy.

Case II reported by Perreau and Rouchy had pruritus followed by jaundice in the 3rd month of her first two pregnancies, both times with premature deliveries in the 6th month and subsidence of jaundice afterwards. During the second pregnancy bilirubinuria was present, serum bilirubin was 19.8 mg per 100 ml (direct-reacting bilirubin 14.9 mg per 100 ml), akaline phosphatase was 8.6 Bodansky units, prothrombin time was normal and the flocculation reactions were negative. A liver biopsy 9 days after delivery showed dislocated hepatic cell plates, enlarged liver cells with clarification of the cytoplasm, hyperplasia of the Kupffer cells and a mild increase in connective tissue. This was interpreted as "diffuse hepatitis". Jaundice disappeared 3 weeks after delivery and she was asymptomatic during the next 4 years. She then became pregnant for the third time and developed pruritus followed by jaundice in the 5th month. Serum bilirubin was 15.8 mg per 100 ml, bilirubinuria was present, and the cephalin flocculation was 1 +. She delivered at 7 1/2 months and jaundice disappeared one week later. Six months after delivery she had a large and firm spleen, a serum bilirubin of 1.5 mg per 100 ml and no excretion of contrast material during radiological gallbladder examination. At present she has the full picture of liver cirrhosis verified by liver biopsy (personal communication from Dr. Perreau).

This case clearly developed toward liver cirrhosis while presenting with jaundice during 3 successive pregnancies. Again, chronic hepatitis is most likely the underlying primary disease.

Another possible example of chronic underlying liver disease after hepatitis with exacerbation during pregnancy is a case published by Puyo (Mme. Le B., observation of Cachera, also published by Caroli et al. and by Lacomme). This woman had viral hepatitis of mild degree at age 22. At age 23 she became icteric during the 4th month of her first pregnancy and had dark urine and light stools. She delivered at 8 1/2 months and jaundice disappeared one month later. During her second pregnancy she became jaundiced in the 4th month, delivered in the 6th and was "cured" one month afterwards. Six months later she had an enlarged firm liver and spleen, a serum bilirubin of 3.2 mg per 100 ml and a positive cephalin flocculation. Liver biopsy showed "hyperplasia of the architecture of the liver cell plates". During her third pregnancy she was again jaundiced before her delivery at term.

Recurrent jaundice of pregnancy due to incipient primary biliary cirrhosis

A case published by Tylecote in 1914 may well represent an example of primary biliary cirrhosis. This woman underwent 8 pregnancies during the age of 18 to 32 years. In each pregnancy there was an insidious onset of jaundice with bilirubinuria during the 3rd month of gestation. She usually delivered prematurely during the 7th or 8th month of gestation and jaundice did not clear until 3 months after delivery. Since the last pregnancy she remained permanently jaundiced, her liver was markedly enlarged and massive xanthomatosis appeared. With the rapid succession of her multiple pregnancies and the long duration of jaundice after delivery it is possible that this woman was more or less permanently jaundiced already before the onset of her xanthomatosis.

No definite diagnosis can be made in this case because eight pregnancies would be very unusual in primary biliary cirrhosis. Ahrens et al. reported 17 females with this disease, 10 of which had an uncomplicated pregnancy prior to the clinical manifestation of their cirrhosis. Three were pregnant during their illness. In two of these bilirubin levels were not followed at that time, while in one there was a sharp drop of serum bilirubin and serum lipids during pregnancy, to rise again after a spontaneous abortion in the 4th month.

Recurrent jaundice during pregnancy due to posthepatitic hyperbilirubinemia

Posthepatic hyperbilirubinemia, thoroughly discussed by Kalk on the basis of 165 cases, is a syndrome indistinguishable from the familial Gilbert's syndrome except for the presence of viral hepatitis in the past history. It is characterized by a mild elevation of the indirect reacting serum bilirubin fraction with a normal direct reacting bilirubin and normal results in all other tests used to evaluate liver function.

Dietel has published a case with posthepatitic hyperbilirubinemia during 2 pregnancies (case E. Fr.). Two years after a first normal pregnancy this woman had typical viral hepatitis. During the next two pregnancies, 2 and 4 years after her hepatitis respectively, she became mildly jaundiced during the last trimester with an elevation of the indirect serum bilirubin to between 2.7 and 3.5 mg per 100 ml. Hemolysis was excluded and all other liver tests were normal. Jaundice disappeared within one week after delivery.

A second case of Dietel's represents posthepatitic hyperbilirubinemia during one pregnancy only. This woman contracted viral hepatitis one year after her first normal pregnancy. Two years after the hepatitis she became pregnant for the second time and developed mild jaundice during the last trimester with elevation of the indirect serum bilirubin fraction to between 2.5 and 3.5 mg per 100 ml. Liver biopsy in this case was normal and jaundice cleared rapidly after delivery. Martini et al. mention three similar cases without giving any details.

Recurrent jaundice during pregnancy
due to gallstones in the common
bile duct
It has already been mentioned that jaundice due to common duct stones is extremely rare during pregnancy. It is not astonishing, therefore, that no documented cases of recurrent jaundice during prenancy due to this condition exist. Two cases may possibly fall into this category. Rissmann described in 1910 a patient with several episodes of biliary colic before her first pregnancy. One week before term during her first pregnancy she had a similar attack followed by jaundice which disappeared after delivery. Jaundice with colicky pains in the right upper abdominal quadrant occurred again two weeks before delivery during her second pregnancy. Another example may be case 1 (Mme. B. S.) reported by Puyo and again by Caroli et al. This woman was jaundiced during the 6th month of her first pregnancy.

Jaundice disappeared after delivery in the 7th month. The patient was plagued with intermittent colicky pains in the gallbladder area ever since. During the next pregnancy she was jaundiced from the 7th month until after her delivery at term. Cholelithiasis was found on radiological examination and a cholecystectomy was performed some months later. During the third pregnancy she had again an episode of jaundice lasting 4 weeks during the 4th month of gestation, but this time it cleared well before delivery.

Recurrent jaundice during pregnancy
due to familial non-hemolytic jaundice
Four cases of this syndrome have been reported in the literature. In all hemolysis has been excluded with a reasonable degree of certitude, but in none an exact diagnosis could be established (such as Gilbert's syndrome, the Rotor syndrome or the Dubin—Johnson syndrome).

Paschkis reports a case with "constitutional hyperbilirubinemia" and jaundice during 12 successive gestations. A case of "Cholémie familiale", published by Chabrol, a pupil of Gilbert, had subicterus and an enlarged spleen when not pregnant and "extremely intensive jaundice" with epistaxis and melena during 3 successive gestations, each time subsiding after spontaneous abortion. Two patients with chronic mild jaundice and a history of the same disorder in their fathers and in one instance in a twin sister are reported by Ikonen. Case E. K. had jaundice with a serum bilirubin of 3.8 mg per 100 ml in her otherwise uncomplicated first pregnancy. The next two pregnancies terminated in spontaneous abortions. The chronic subicterus deepened again during the 4th gestation, the patient developed some epigastric pain and the liver margin became palpable and tender. There was no bilirubinuria and the thymol turbidity was negative. A bromsulfalein clearance was interpreted as "pointing to the Dubin—Johnson syndrome". Liver biopsy was refused and a cholecystogram normal. Case H. F. with chronic subicterus had first an abortion in the 3rd month. During the second pregnancy the serum bilirubin was 2.6 mg per 100 ml and no bilirubin was present in the urine. She aborted in the 5th month. In the third pregnancy serum bilirubin was 2.0 mg per 100 ml, alkaline phosphatase 4.3 Bessey—Lowry units and SGOT 59 units. Urine bilirubin was negative. Premature delivery took place in the 7th month. One year later the patient became febrile and jaundiced. Radiological examination revealed gall stones.

Recurrent jaundice during pregnancy due to hemolysis

Two examples of hemolysis with jaundice due to unknown cause are reported in the literature. The first seven pregnancies in the case of Bromberg et al. were uncomplicated. During the 8th gestation headache, dizziness, anorexia and jaundice were noted in the 7th month. Hemoglobin was 6.1 mg per 100 ml, reticulocyte counts markedly elevated and total serum bilirubin 2.2 mg per 100 ml with a negative direct Van den Bergh reaction. Urine bilirubin was absent and urobilinogen increased. The woman de-

livered at term and recovered rapidly thereafter. During the next four years no acute hemolytic crisis occurred, but her hemoglobin remained around 7.5 to 9 gm per 100 ml, reticulocyte counts remained elevated and the spleen became enlarged. She became pregnant for the 9th time and suffered from an acute hemolytic crisis in the 25th week, with a drop in hemoglobin to 4.5 gm per 100 ml and a rise in serum bilirubin to 4.6 mg per 100 ml. After induced abortion she recovered rapidly. Radiological gallbladder examination was normal.

The case of Zachariae had a normal first pregnancy, followed by one with an abortion. She was anemic during her third gestation (hemoglobin 51 %). Towards the end of her 4th pregnancy the hemoglobin dropped to 37 % and jaundice with a serum bilirubin of 5.0 mg per 100 ml was present until delivery 3 weeks later. Splenomegaly was noted. During the next 2 years she had once a hemolytic episode without jaundice while suffering from thrombophlebitis. During the fifth pregnancy hemolysis with jaundice occurred in the third month and was cured by an induced abortion.

A third case of recurrent jaundice during pregnancy is due to congenital spherocytosis (Rimbach and Beickert). The patient's father, the father's brother and mother had chronic mild jaundice, while the patient herself was never jaundiced outside her pregnancies. During 4 consecutive gestations she developed hemolytic crisis with jaundice, the hemoglobin dropping each time to about 30 %. Each time hemolysis disappeared within 2 weeks after delivery. The spleen was enlarged and morphological blood examination was consistent with spherocytosis.

A fourth case, reported by Schneider and Frahm, has a mixed etiology. This woman had anemia during her 3rd and 4th pregnancy, and hemolytic anemia with mild jaundice during her 5th and 6th pregnancy. Investigation revealed a large spleen and a megaloblastic bone marrow. After the cure of her pernicious anemia with Vitamin B 12 the red cell morphology was typical for congenital spherocytosis, which subsequently was discovered to exist also in 3 of her siblings.

Recurrent jaundice with hemoglobinuria during pregnancy

In 1902 both Schaeffer and Brauer reported the case of an Italian woman with marked pruritus and mild jaundice in the second half of 6 successive pregnancies except during the third which was terminated early by a spontaneous abortion. General symptoms were mild and the jaundice cleared rapidly after delivery. The dark urine contained bilirubin, urobilin and in addition hemoglobin. A similar non-recurrent case was observed by Meinhold in 1903 in a primipara, with marked pruritus and hemoglobinuria, but without jaundice and without bile constituents in the urine. Both patients inhabited areas were malaria was common, both had no fever and both had negative tests for malaria.

No further case of pregnancy with hemoglobinuria has been reported since. It is therefore unlikely that such an entity exists in reality.

Recurrent jaundice during pregnancy due to severe pyelonephritis

The only acceptable case of recurrent jaundice during pregnancy due to pyelonephritis in the literature is the one published by Fruhinsholz in 1929. During the 4th month of her first pregnancy this woman developed fever, chills, pains in the right flank, anorexia and vomiting, followed by oliguria. In the 5th month, while fever continued, frank jaundice was observed with a large and tender liver. Massive pyuria continued. Purpura developed on the extremities. An induced abortion was performed and the woman recovered rapidly. During the 7th month of the second pregnancy there was again pyuria, dysuria, pollacisuria and finally oliguria, shortly followed by jaundice with a large tender liver. This time there was no temperature elevation. The woman delivered 2 weeks later and jaundice disappeared rapidly.

Since the advent of sulfonamides and antibiotics no similar cases have been observed.

Recurrent jaundice during pregnancy due to hyperemesis gravidarum

A well-documented case of this disorder is presented by Thorling (case 33). This woman had hyperemesis during her first pregnancy without jaundice and developed pruritus during the last month of gestation. During the second pregnancy she had again marked hyperemesis starting in the 11th week, followed shortly by itching, dark urine and manifest jaundice. There was urobilinuria, no bilirubinuria, an increase in serum bilirubin and alkaline phosphatase and a normal thymol turbidity. Upon hospitalisation the symptoms subsided rapidly and she delivered without further complications at term. During the next pregnancy she had again hyperemesis, this time lasting during her whole gestation, with intermittent episodes of dark urine and jaundice. Pruritus developed during the last two months. Upon delivery she became immediately symptomfree.

Another possible example is the case reported by Lantuéjoul and Chambraud. This woman had hepatitis at 12 years of age. During her first two pregnancies she suffered from marked hyperemesis without jaundice and delivered prematurely both times. The sequence of events was the same in her third pregnancy, but this time dark urine and jaundice were noted before delivery in the 7th month. During the 4th pregnancy hyperemesis started in the 6th month and jaundice in the 7th. Bilirubin and urobilin were present in the urine, serum bilirubin rose to 5.7 mg per 100 ml, the thymol turbidity and the cephalin flocculation were positive. After delivery a few weeks later she rapidly recovered.

There are no reported cases with detailed laboratory data and in none has a liver biopsy been performed (see also page 39). Jaundice due to hyperemesis is clearly distinct from intrahepatic cholestasis of pregnancy by the presence of vomiting and by its cure well before delivery.

Recurrent jaundice during pregnancy with different etiology of jaundice in successive pregnancies

Three case reports will illustrate the diagnostic difficulties encountered in some cases of recurrent jaundice during pregnancy. In these, jaundice of different origin occurred in successive pregnancies, or jaundice was of mixed etiology.

Case 16 reported by Nixon et al. had an abortion during the 6th week of her first gestation. In the 20th week of her second pregnancy she developed anorexia, nausea and vomiting, then dark urine and light stools followed by frank jaundice in the 24th week. Liver and spleen were enlarged, serum bilirubin rose to 18.2 mg per 100 ml and liver biopsy revealed typical acute viral hepatitis. She delivered in the 30th week and jaundice cleared only within 2—3 months. Five months later a liver biopsy was normal. One and a half years later she was again pregnant. During the 5th month she became icteric. The total serum bilirubin was 3.4 mg per 100 ml with normal amounts of the direct reacting fraction, and hemoglobin dropped to 45 %. In the 7th month total bilirubin was 1.4 mg per 100 ml. While this patient had proved viral hepatitis during the second pregnancy it appears probable that she had hemolytic jaundice during the third.

Less clear is a case reported by Ezès and Bourdon. This woman was jaundiced from the 5th month until term in her first two pregnancies and jaundice cleared rapidly after delivery. Jaundice again became apparent in the 6th month of her 3rd pregnancy. Examinations at that time revealed a total serum bilirubin of 9.4 mg per 100 ml (direct reacting 6.4 mg per 100 ml), a low serum cholesterol, a prolonged prothrombin time, and an increase of gamma globulins to 33 % on electrophoresis.

She had a hematocrit of 36 % and a reticulocyte count of 6 %. Here, hemolysis appears to be an additional factor to whatever was the primary disease, which could have been chronic hepatitis or cirrhosis of the liver.

A similar case has been observed by Lebon et al. During the first two pregnancies this woman was jaundiced from the 7th month until shortly after her deliveries in the 8th month. During her third pregnancy she developed asthenia and pruritus in the 5th month, followed by intense arthralgias, back and chest pains, and then by jaundice. The liver was enlarged and tender, her general health markedly impaired, with a weight loss of 13 kg. Bilirubinuria was present, total serum bilirubin was 2.4 mg per 100 ml, alkaline phosphatase 15.8 Bodansky units, the flocculation reactions normal, serum cholesterol low, and liver biopsy showed a granular degeneration of the liver cells, an increase in Kupffer cells and an increase in reticulum. This was interpreted as "periportal hepatitis". Her red cell count was 2,700,000 per cu. mm and reticulocytes were 3.4 %, so that hemolysis appears superimposed to what was — from the history — viral hepatitis during her 3rd pregnancy. The episodes of jaundice during her first two pregnancies are not explained. Hypothetically it is possible that a woman has recurrent intrahepatic cholestasis during two pregnancies and then viral hepatitis during the third.

Recurrent jaundice during pregnancy due to unclassified causes

Five cases of recurrent jaundice during pregnancy cannot be classified at all.

Two sisters with recurrent jaundice during pregnancy were reported by both Benedict and Lovrich. Pruritus and jaundice occurred in case 1 during 4, in case 2 during 2 gestations. In both cases onset of jaundice was in the first trimester. During the fourth pregnancy of case 1 the liver and the spleen were markedly enlarged and hard, during the second pregnancy of case 2 the liver was enlarged and the spleen was not palpable but enlarged to percussion. Cirrhosis of the liver or a familial hemolytic disorder (urine constantly negative for bilirubin) are not excluded in these cases.

The case described by Vignes in 1935 with jaundice during the 7th to 10th pregnancies has been considered to represent hemolytic jaundice by the author. The patient had tachycardia, dyspnoe, oliguria and pruritus besides jaundice, and looked "increasingly toxic". Not enough details are given to permit a retrospective evaluation.

Case 19 of Nixon et al. was jaundiced from the 24th week until delivery at term in her first pregnancy. Jaundice appeared again in the 10th week of her second pregnancy. The liver was enlarged and total serum bilirubin rose to 10.5 mg per 100 ml. Two liver biopsies were performed, both showing hyperplasia of the Kupffer cells and a fair amount of biliary pigment in the reticulum cells. The patient was not followed. In this case a hemolytic disorder or a subsiding viral hepatitis may be considered.

Case II of Boquien et al. was jaundiced during the 2nd, 3rd and 4th pregnancy. During the second pregnancy eclampsia with hypertension and protein-uria occurred during the 8th month, followed by jaundice, convulsions, and delivery of a stillborn child by Caesarian section. During the 8th month of the 3rd pregnancy hypertension was observed and then delivery of a stillborn child took place in the presence of a retroplacentar hematoma. Jaundice began at delivery and lasted for some weeks. Hemolysis was excluded. During the fourth pregnancy — again complicated by hypertension — pruritus and jaundice began one day after Caesarian section in the 8th month, lasting for 10 days. As jaundice began *after* delivery in the last two gestations, intrahepatic cholestasis of pregnancy seems excluded. Eclampsia appears to have caused jaundice during the second and possibly also during the 3rd pregnancy.

The case reported by Justin—Besançon et al. had onset of pruritus and jaundice during the first month of her first pregnancy, associated with vomiting. She delivered at term and jaundice disappeared two weeks later. General health was markedly impaired and she lost 10 kg body weight during her gestation. During her second gestation jaundice and pruritus appeared in the 7th week after a prodromal phase of anorexia and vomiting. Because of impaired general condition and weight loss of 5 kg abortion was induced in the 12th week. This resulted in fever up to 38° centigrade and in an increase in jaundice. Twelve days later her serum bilirubin was 18.0 mg per 100 ml. Three weeks after delivery serum bilirubin was 3.5 mg per 100 ml with positive reactions to the thymol turbidity and the

zinc sulfate flocculation. Peritoneoscopy on the 31st day after delivery was unremarkable, bromsulfalein retention on the 37th day was 45 % after 45 minutes, a liver biopsy on the 43rd day (2 weeks after subsidence of jaundice) showed minimal cholestasis, and radiological gallbladder examination was normal. The general symptoms and weight loss, as well as the intensity of jaundice would point towards viral hepatitis as the cause of jaundice during the second gestation, but this cannot be conclusively proved.

Misquoted cases of recurrent jaundice during pregnancy in the literature

The case of Bjerregaard, published in 1904, had 3 normal pregnancies, then three with pruritus alone, followed by pruritus and jaundice during the 7th gestation only. This case is repeatedly cited as representing recurrent jaundice during pregnancy. In these quotations the author's name is usually mis-spelled and the bibliography incomplete or incorrect. Most likely few reviewers bothered to have the Danish original translated.

Another case often quoted is one published in a French journal in 1907 by M. L. A. Meyer. The case report is truly an example of recurrent jaundice during pregnancy, but represents only a French abstract of a German paper by A. Mayer in 1906 with the author's name mis-spelled. Among the author's initials in the French abstract the M. stands for "monsieur" and the origin of the L. cannot be traced.

A case of Enrile et al. with tuberculoma of the liver has been called recurrent jaundice occasionally. This

TABLE 23. Recurrent jaundice *during* pregnancy

A. Recurrent jaundice *in* pregnancy

I. Recurrent jaundice recurring also in non-pregnant subjects
  1. Recurrent viral hepatitis or exacerbation of anicteric chronic hepatitis
  2. Recurrent jaundice in primary biliary cirrhosis
  3. Recurrent posthepatitic hyperbilirubinemia
  4. Recurrent common bile duct obstruction due to gall stones
  5. Recurrent exacerbations of familial non-hemolytic jaundice
  6. Recurrent hemolytic jaundice
  7. Recurrent jaundice with hemoglobinuria (??)

II. Recurrent jaundice due to medical complications of pregnancy
  1. Recurrent jaundice in severe pyelonephritis

B. Recurrent jaundice *of* pregnancy

I. Recurrent idiopathic jaundice of pregnancy
  1. Recurrent intrahepatic cholestasis of pregnancy
II. Recurrent jaundice as complication of disease linked to pregnancy
  1. Recurrent jaundice in hyperemesis gravidarum

C. Recurrent jaundice during pregnancy due to different diseases causing jaundice during pregnancy
  Example: Hepatitis in one, hemolytic jaundice in the other gestation

D. Non-classified cases of recurrent jaundice during pregnancy

woman had 3 episodes of jaundice during a single pregnancy (her fifth).

4) Classification of recurrent jaundice during pregnancy

A classification of recurrent jaundice during pregnancy based on the cases described in chapter III/2 and III/3 is given in Table 23. The same general subdivisions are used as in Table 3 in the classification of (non-recurrent) jaundice during pregnancy. It is theoretically possible, that other diseases listed in Table 3 and not listed in Table 23 could be recurrent, such as jaundice due to toxemia of pregnancy or jaundice due to tetracycline toxicity. We have refrained from listing them under re-

current jaundice during pregnancy before actual cases with adequate documentation are presented.

5) Other diseases with recurrent jaundice and complete recovery in the anicteric interval

Many patients with chronic liver disease such as chronic hepatitis or cirrhosis of the liver may run a course characterized by periods of exacerbations with jaundice and relatively symptom-free anicteric intervals. Residual functional and/or structural damage persists, however, in these diseases. Apart from recurrent intrahepatic cholestasis of pregnancy only one disease is at present known with recurrent jaundice and complete recovery in the anicteric intervals. It shall be briefly mentioned, mainly to show that its course differs markedly in all other respects from that seen in intrahepatic cholestasis of pregnancy. Another, probably non-existing entity referred to in the older literature shall be listed to complete this survey.

Idiopathic recurrent cholestasis

Of this curious and only recently discovered disease only 12 cases have so far been described (Summerskill and Walshe 1959 2 cases, Tygstrup 1960 2 cases, De Groote et al. 1960 2 cases, Kühn 1960 2 cases, Schapiro and Isselbacher 1963 1 case and Williams et al. 1964 3 cases). The entity consists of recurrent episodes of intrahepatic obstructive jaundice with complete clinical, functional and histological recovery in the intervals. Two patients are females and 10 are males. Two patients are brothers (Kühn), two adolescent males are possibly related (Tygstrup) and in the other eight the family history is negative. First symptoms occurred between the ages of 1 and 29 years, with 5 patients in the first, 4 in the second and 3 in the third decade. The longest observed duration after the first attack of jaundice is 37 years, with 27 episodes of jaundice recorded (Schapiro and Isselbacher).

An attack starts usually with a mild prodromal syndrome of anorexia and fatigue of up to 2 weeks' duration. Marked pruritus and jaundice then set in, lasting usually around 4 months with a range from 1 to 10 months. There is no fever or pain. Steatorrhea (up to 48 gm fecal fat excretion per day (Tygstrup case 2)) during jaundice leads to a marked weight loss, despite good appetite. Weight loss is always regained in the asymptomatic interval. Jaundice is usually accompanied by moderate hepatomegaly. The spleen was slightly enlarged in two cases. Chemically, an "obstructive pattern" is observed. Serum bilirubin levels are usually between 8 and 23 mg per 100 ml, but may reach 40 mg per 100 ml. Serum alkaline phosphatase is mildly to moderately elevated, but may attain 94 King—Armstrong units. Serum cholesterol, however, is usually normal. It was mildly elevated in 2 cases (Tygstrup) and reached 380 mg per 100 ml in the case which also presents the highest recorded levels for serum bilirubin and alkaline phosphatase (Schapiro and Isselbacher). Serum transaminases have been normal or only slightly elevated. Serum turbidity and flocculation tests are normal as well as the albumin/globulin ratio. The erythrocyte sedimentation rate is slightly elevated and electrophoresis shows a mild increase in alpha-2 and beta-globulins (Kühn, Williams et al.). Intravenous bilirubin tolerance tests show a regurgitation of conjugated bilirubin from the liver cells into the blood stream during jaundice, but are normal in the anicteric interval (Williams et al.). Gallbladder X-rays usually show no filling during jaundice, but all intraoperative cholangiograms have been normal.

Liver biopsies during jaundice show marked centrolobular bile stasis with bile plugs in the canaliculi and bile pigment in the hepatocytes and in the Kupffer cells. In the centrolobular areas there is hepatocellular degeneration, loss of liver cells and inflammatory infiltration. Some portal tracts show edema or infiltration (Williams et al.). Biopsies in anicteric intervals are normal or may show minimal residual bile stasis. Laparatomies and peritoneoscopies have revealed a brownish or greenish discoloration of the liver but otherwise normal findings.

Both of the 2 reported women have been pregnant during the course of their disease. The case with 27 episodes of jaundice during age 3 and 40 underwent a single normal anicteric pregnancy at age 25 (Schapiro and Isselbacher). The other woman had her first episode of jaundice in the second month of her first pregnancy. After an artificial abortion in the fourth month of gestation the jaundice persisted. Three further pregnancies were anicteric during the whole course.

Thus, pregnancy does not induce a relapse of jaundice in this disease.

Recurrent jaundice during menstruation

In 1872 Senator described 4 women who developed jaundice for a few days during each successive menstrual bleeding. A careful review of his case reports does not support his enthusiastic association of jaundice with menstruation. The maximal episodes of jaundice in a single patient were six, with anicteric menstruations or — in one case — a normal pregnancy thereafter. Furthermore the time relationship is not always convincing. During the "disease" jaundice is said to occur instead of a missed menstrual bleeding. From the data presented it is impossible to diagnose the nature of this jaundice. A fifth case in the litera-

ture, reported by Metzger in 1904, is clearly a description of an acute viral hepatitis with several relapses.

No further such cases have been described and it must be concluded that "recurrent jaundice during menstruation" does not exist.

6) Pathogenesis of intrahepatic cholestasis of pregnancy

A review of the older literature concerning speculations on the pathogenesis of recurrent jaundice during pregnancy has been presented by Mayer in 1906. The prevalent idea at that time was a mechanical compression of the extrahepatic bile ducts by the enlarged uterus pressing on a constipated transverse colon. This mirrors the views held by the authors of textbooks on liver disease in the 19th century (Budd and Henoch 1846, Frerichs 1858, Quincke and Hoppe—Seyler 1899). Other theories on the pathogenesis of benign jaundice during pregnancy included "nervous influences", "plethora of organs during pregnancy", "dyspepsia", "gastroduodenitis", a "mucous plug in the common bile duct" and "sudden emotions" (Meunier 1872).

A similar line of thought is persued by Roumanian authors in 1957 (Pavel et al.) who assume that distension of the peritoneum overlying the enlarging uterus triggers nervous reflexes which then will — modified by a terrain of hyperfolliculinemia — lead to a spasm of the sphincter of Oddi and perhaps to reflex inhibition of bile secretion.

Early in the 20th century most authors were convinced of a causal relationship between pregnancy and recurrent jaundice (Kehrer 1905), but some still denied a connection vehemently (Schickele 1910) or believed these cases to be due to gallstone obstruction (Rissmann 1910).

Gallstone obstruction of the common bile duct as a cause of cholestasis of pregnancy has been excluded since radiological examination of the gallbladder has been possible. Ikonen considers the incidence of coincidental gall stones not causing obstruction high in intrahepatic cholestasis of pregnancy (this opinion is based on non-recurrent cases) and believes that gall stone formation could well be explained as a parallel phenomenon arising from the same disorder in metabolism which is causing the clinical picture of "obstetric hepatosis".

With the recognition of viral hepatitis as one of the most common liver diseases during World War II the causal relationship between pregnancy and recurrent jaundice was questioned again and many, especially French authors considered the disorder to represent a recurrence or exacerbation of a previous viral hepatitis under the stress of pregnancy. The arguments for or against such a viewpoint have been summarized by Caroli et al. in 1954, who concluded that recurrent jaundice of pregnancy will but rarely be caused by viral hepatitis.

A type of latent familial non-hemolytic jaundice with manifestation during pregnancy is suggested by the familial occurrence of intrahepatic cholestasis of pregnancy in at least 6 instances (see page 70). Gilbert's syndrome with an elevation of the indirect serum bilirubin fraction only is ruled out immediately. Both the Rotor and the Dubin—Johnson syndrome have an elevation of the direct-reacting bilirubin fraction. In the Dubin—Johnson syndrome pruritus is usually absent and the alkaline phosphatase not elevated. Liver biopsy with the characteristic blackbrown pigment is quite different from liver biopsy in intrahepatic cholestasis of pregnancy (Dubin). Liver biopsy in the Rotor syndrome is normal, as it is in some cases of intrahepatic cholestasis of pregnancy. Laboratory findings are somewhat similar, but bromsulfalein retention is more pronounced and oral contrast materials visualize the gallbladder well. The patients with the Rotor syndrome are asymptomatic and do not have pruritus (Schiff et al., Peck et al.). Furthermore jaundice decreases during pregnancy (Haverback and Wirtschafter).

The concept of "bile stasis" was probably first advanced by Boreel in 1924. It was clearly expressed by Perreau in 1953 and by Svanborg in 1954. Thorling in 1955 proposed the concept of "incomplete intrahepatic biliary tract obstruction precipitated by hepatic damage". The main theories advanced to explain the mechanism of intrahepatic cholestasis in this disorder are: atony of the extrahepatic biliary passages (Svanborg), change in the chemical composition of bile leading to inspissation (Ljunggren) and a change in membrane permeability at the level of the bile capillaries (Gros). The first two possibilities appear unlikely because of the observation of normal bile drainage from a T-tube in the case of Béraud et al. This provides of course no evidence in favour of the membrane permeability theory.

Whenever the etiology of a disease is unknown, one is inclined to draw analogies to similar diseases. The syndrome "intrahepatic cholestasis" includes (apart from pregnancy) viral hepatitis, drug-induced cholestasis, acute fatty liver and alcoholism (Dölle and Martini 1959 and 1962, Jeffries and Sleisenger).

Fatty liver and alcoholism can readily be excluded on the basis of liver biopsy findings and personal history in patients with intrahepatic cholestasis of pregnancy.

Viral hepatitis may occur under the form of pure intrahepatic cholestasis without signs of inflammation or liver cell damage on liver biopsy (Caroli et al. 1953, Dubin et al. 1960, histological type D). These cases are extremely rare (6 patients in these two papers) and present clinically the usual prodromal symptoms seen in typical acute viral hepatitis, which are absent in intrahepatic cholestasis of pregnancy. More frequent are forms of viral hepatitis with obstructive features (so-called "cholangiolitic hepatitis") with findings of typical viral hepatitis on biopsy (Watson and Hoffbauer, Gall and Braunstein, Dubin et al., histological types B and C) so that they are easily distinguishable from intrahepatic cholestasis of pregnancy.

Primary biliary cirrhosis may in the initial stages present with pruritus without jaundice, with an elevation of alkaline phosphatase and an elevation of bromsulfalein retention (Popper et al. 1962). No case of recurrent cholestasis of pregnancy has yet progressed to primary biliary cirrhosis. The case reported by Tylecote probably represented primary biliary cirrhosis from the onset of its clinical course.

Drug-induced cholestasis is most likely to induce comparison with intrahepatic cholestasis of pregnancy, especially as sex hormones can be implicated in both disorders. In addition, Read et al. suggested that pregnant women may be especially susceptible to the development of chlorpromazine-induced jaundice, although this has not been confirmed by others (see page 32).

Drug-induced intrahepatic cholestasis consists of two main types: a sensitivity type (example chlorpromazine-jaundice) which histologically shows portal infiltrations in addition to cholestasis, and a non-sensitivity type (example norethandrolone-jaundice) with the histological picture of pure cholestasis (Sherlock). The latter type is histologically comparable to intrahepatic cholestasis of pregnancy. It is produced by methyltestosterone and other C-17-α-alkyl-substituted testosterones, such as norethandrolone (Nilevar®), methandienone (Dianabol®) and the ovulation inhibitor Enavid® which contains norethynodrel.

In this connection an interesting observation has been made in case L. A. reported by Ikonen. This woman with intrahepatic cholestasis of pregnancy in 2 successive gestations was given an ovulation inhibitor containing norethisterone and aethinyloestradiol 9 1/2 months after the last delivery. She developed abdominal pains, nausea and — after one week — dark urine and pruritus, followed by jaundice and an increase in

SGOT. The drug was stopped and jaundice disappeared. The patient later received progesterone without ill effect.

King and Kerrins, in their report on a case with recurrent intrahepatic cholestasis of pregnancy, considered this disorder to have a "striking resemblance to drug-induced jaundice". Similar opinions have been voiced by Svanborg and Ohlsson and by Gros. Such statements have to be firmly refused. Although the case of Ikonen suggests that pregnancy and the ovulation-inhibitor triggered the same disease process and although histology in norethandrolone-type cholestasis is indistinguishable from intrahepatic cholestasis of pregnancy, there are important and mutually exclusive differences between the two disorders. Jaundice in intrahepatic cholestasis of pregnancy is always mild and is not known to have surpassed a serum bilirubin level of 8.4 mg per 100 ml. In drug-induced cholestasis jaundice is mild in the majority of cases, but may reach levels of up to 30 mg per 100 ml of serum bilirubin (Werner et al). In norethandrolone-type jaundice alkaline phosphatase is comparatively little elevated. Furthermore, a prodromal period with anorexia, malaise and often fever is common in drug-induced jaundice (Schaffner) and was present in the ovulation inhibitor-induced jaundice in Ikonen's case, while prodromi are absent in intrahepatic cholestasis of pregnancy. In addition, pruritus is the dominant symptom in intrahepatic cholestasis of pregnancy, while in drug-induced jaundice pruritus is present in only about half the cases. More significant even, methyltestosterone and norethandrolone are effective therapeutic agents to relieve pruritus of hepatic origin, although they increase the intensity of pre-existing jaundice at the same time.

A disordered hormonal balance remains an attractive hypothesis for the basic pathogenetic mechanism in intrahepatic cholestasis of pregnancy, but such a hypothesis should not be founded on a comparison of this disease with steroid-induced jaundice as we know it at present. ·

It might be worth while to consider briefly the meaning of the term "intrahepatic cholestasis". Cholestasis has been given two basic definitions: a clinical-functional one and a histological one. Clinically and functionally cholestasis is defined as a disease with pruritus, an elevation of serum alkaline phosphatase and often an elevation of serum cholesterol. Histologically cholestasis is defined as the presence of bile plugs (or bile thrombi) in the bile canaliculi (or bile capillaries), and the presence of bile pigment in hepatic cells and Kupffer cells predominantly in the centrolobular area (Popper and Schaffner). While in most examples of intrahepatic cholestasis functional and histological cholestasis are present more or less parallel to one another, in others they are not and functional or histological cholestasis may be completely absent. On one end of this spectrum lies the entity called "postoperative intrahepatic cholestasis" which presents a marked and pure cholestasis on liver biopsies but functionally predominantly an elevation of serum bilirubin of up to 27 mg per 100 ml with normal or mildly elevated alkaline phosphatase and absence of pruritus (Schmid et al.). Intrahepatic cholestasis of pregnancy represents the other end of this spectrum, as in this disorder pruritus is violent, biochemical cholestasis usually impressive and histological cholestasis focal and minimal, so minimal that it can be easily missed by the pathologist. At present no explanation can be offered for this divergence of functional and structural cholestasis, but this aspect should be kept in mind when pathogenesis is discussed.

An explanation of the pathogenesis of recurrent intrahepatic cholestasis of pregnancy has — in order to be of value — to explain all of the following features in this disorder:

1. The disorder is strictly linked to pregnancy and does not occur in non-pregnant subjects.
2. The disorder usually presents as "jaundice during late pregnancy" although onset of jaundice may be as early as in the first trimester in some cases.
3. Pruritus is the first symptom to occur and the main symptom during the course of the disease.
4. Apart from pruritus there are no prodromal symptoms. There is a conspicuous absence of general symptoms such as fever, weakness, malaise, anorexia, nausea, vomiting, dyspepsia, pains, colics, arthralgias, weight loss.
5. Jaundice is always of mild degree. The highest observed serum bilirubin level is 8.4 mg per 100 ml. In most cases it is below 6 mg per 100 ml. Direct-reacting bilirubin constitutes the main portion of total serum bilirubin elevation. Bilirubin-

uria is transient or intermittent, but probably present in all cases.
6. Serum alkaline phosphatase and serum cholesterol are elevated in most and serum transaminases in many cases. Any of these three parameters may occasionally be normal in a single patient. Highest observed values are: alkaline phosphatase 28 Bodansky units, serum cholesterol 590 mg per 100 ml, SGOT 920 units, SGPT 875 units (although transaminases are with few exception below 250 units). Serum electrophoresis shows an increase in alpha 2- and mainly in beta-globulins, with normal or slightly decreased gamma-globulins. There is no correlation between any two laboratory tests.
7. Bromsulfalein retention is increased and galactose tolerance is normal. Bromsulfalein clearance studies reveal a decreased hepatic storage capacity and an increased cholestatic index.
8. Rapid improvement sets in after delivery, whether delivery is spontaneous or induced.
9. In closely followed cases there may be a transient return to normal of serum bilirubin and of transaminases on the first postpartum day.
10. Recovery after delivery is complete. No permanent liver damage ensues after multiple pregnancies with jaundice.
11. Histological cholestasis on liver biopsy is mild and focal or irregular. This is in marked contrast to the impressive clinical and biochemical signs of cholestasis.

12. Drainage of bile from a T-tube in the common bile duct is normal during jaundice.
13. Premature delivery is frequent, but limited to some women, while about two thirds of the patients deliver at term. There is no correlation between premature delivery and any other feature of the disorder.
14. The intensity of symptoms during successive pregnancies with jaundice may remain equal, may increase or may decrease.
15. Recurrent pruritus gravidarum may be observed before recurrent pruritus with jaundice in some cases.

At present no pathogenetic explanation based on facts can be offered, at least none giving an insight into whatever process launches the disorder. It appears reasonable, however, to assume that — whatever this triggering process is — *physiological derangement of liver function in normal pregnancy, pruritus gravidarum and intrahepatic cholestasis of pregnancy are but three increasing grades of manifestation of the same basic disorder linked in some way to pregnancy* (Friedberg 1951).

In uncomplicated pregnancies there is towards term an increase in alkaline phosphatase, serum cholesterol, serum lipids, alpha- and beta-globulins and bromsulfalein retention, and a decrease in bromsulfalein excretory capacity (BSB T_m) and intravenous bilirubin tolerance. In pruritus gravidarum these same alterations are more pronounced and additionally the serum transaminases are mildly elevated. Intrahepatic cholestasis of pregnancy shows again an increase of the disturbances seen in pruritus gravidarum with the addition of an elevated serum bilirubin, a radiologically non-visualized gallbladder and histological evidence of intrahepatic cholestasis.

Thus, intrahepatic cholestasis of pregnancy is best viewed as an exaggeration of the alterations of liver function occurring to a minor degree also in uncomplicated pregnancies.

SUMMARY

The main purpose of this review is to define the entity called "recurrent intrahepatic cholestasis of pregnancy" and to establish a differential diagnosis on the many disorders which may present as recurrent jaundice during pregnancy.

PART I contains a review on "liver function" during uncomplicated pregnancy. The liver performs its function well during gestation, but most so-called "liver function tests" show some minor deviations from the accepted normal in non-pregnant subjects. These "physiological" derangements are more common in the later weeks of pregnancy and are rapidly rectified after delivery.

Liver biopsy findings remain generally within normal limits. Some minor nonspecific changes may occur, such as a difference in size of liver cells, an increase in size of their nuclei, some irregularities of the nuclei, an increase in bi-nucleated cells, an increased glycogen content of the cytoplasm and occasionally mild lymphocytic infiltrations in the portal tracts.

Spider angiomas and palmar erythema may be found in up to two thirds of pregnant females. These skin changes are rarely impressive.

Liver blood flow remains quantitatively unchanged. As plasma volume and total blood volume increase by about 50 % in normal pregnancy relative liver blood flow (as fraction of cardiac output) decreases somewhat.

Hemoglobin falls as a result of increasing plasma volume. Serum iron fluctuates, but remains on the whole constant. Total white cell counts may be increased to up to 15,000 per cu. mm and a "shift to the left" is not uncommon.

Alkaline phosphatase increases towards term, with usually a pronounced rise after the 7th month of gestation. Serum cholesterol and serum lipids follow the same trend. On electrophoresis a slight increase in alpha-2 and beta globulins is noted. These changes, though mild, are indicative of an "obstructive pattern" even in normal pregnancy.

Serum bilirubin may in a rare case be elevated to up to 2 mg per 100 ml and abnormal urinary bile pigments may be occasionally present. These changes are not related to the stage of pregnancy, in contrast to the "obstructive features" which tend to increase towards term.

Total serum proteins and serum albumin decrease towards term. The flocculation and turbidity tests are usually normal, but positive results are seen in varying proportions of cases, probably dependent more on the technique used in a specific laboratory than on the test itself.

Bromsulfalein retention is slightly increased towards term, due to an increase in hepatic storage capacity and a decrease in maximal excretory capacity. Galactose tolerance remains normal.

The only "liver function tests" to remain normal throughout pregnancy are the serum transaminases and the prothrombin time.

With the exception of the changes in the white cell count most deviations from the normal are minor. Main diagnostic difficulties will be encountered with the alkaline phosphatase and the turbidity or flocculation tests.

PART II contains a review on all diseases causing jaundice *during* pregnancy. Jaundice occurs in about 1 out of every 1,500 gestations, an incidence of 0.067 %. At least 41 % of all cases with jaundice are due to viral hepatitis, and about 21 % due to intrahepatic cholestasis of pregnancy. Common bile duct obstruction accounts for less than 6 % of all cases with jaundice.

A classification of jaundice *during* pregnancy is proposed in Table 3.

A first group of diseases, "jaundice *in* pregnancy", consists of entities seen also in non-pregnant persons, occurring by chance during gestation.

Viral hepatitis during pregnancy has often been quoted to run a severe cause during pregnancy. A review of the literature reveals that pregnant women are not more susceptable to viral hepatitis than non-pregnant subjects, that viral hepatitis runs the same course in pregnancy as outside of it, and that mortality from viral hepatitis is not increased during pregnancy, at least not in Europe. An exception to this rule may be seen in the indigene population of underdeveloped countries, where malnutrition and general debility provide a serious hazard to any additional injury during gestation. Viral hepatitis occurs probably with equal frequency during all trimesters of gestation and not predominantly towards term, as has been frequently stated. The course of severe hepatitis is not influenced by an induced interruption, and termination of pregnancy is not advised. Hepatitis induces an increased incidence of premature deliveries. Child survival depends on the degree of maturity. No conclusive evidence exists that viral hepatitis can be transmitted from the mother to the unborn child, at least not in the later part of gestation.

Pregnancy occurs rarely during cirrhosis of the liver, because fertilization is impaired in this disease. For this reason, cirrhotics who do get pregnant probably represent a selection of the less severe cases and generally tolerate gestation surprisingly well, even when they previously had manifestations of decompensated liver function. Pregnancy increases intra-abdominal pressure and probably also pre-existing portal hypertension. A rare case will develop ascites. Occasionally hematemesis from esophageal varices is induced. Successful porto-caval shunts have been performed during pregnancy. Hematemesis towards terms may be stopped by a Caesarian section. Child survival is not affected by the mother's cirrhosis.

Drug-induced intrahepatic cholestasis (usually due to chlorpromazine) is probably not influenced by pregnancy, although 4 of 22 chronic cases in the literature began in pregnancy, including the case with the longest recorded duration of 3 years before complete recovery. The prodromal phase is similar to that seen in viral hepatitis, the biochemical data show an "obstructive pattern".

Gallstone disease is — contrary to general opinion — in most likelyhood not caused by nor increased during pregnancy and common bile duct obstruction is rare during gestation. It is handled according to general medical or surgical principles.

Data on the behaviour of chronic idiopathic hyperbilirubinemias are sparse. Pregnancy generally aggravates the intensity of jaundice in the Dubin—Johnson syndrome, may lessen it in the Rotor syndrome, and does usually not influence the course in Gilbert's syndrome.

Hemolytic disorders during pregnancy usually present as marked anemia and an accompanying jaundice is generally mild. The primary hemolytic disorders during pregnancy — megaloblastic anemia of pregnancy due to folic acid deficiency and idiopathic hemolysis of pregnancy — are exceedingly rare. Pre-existing chronic hemolytic states may be aggravated during gestation, such as familial spherocytosis and some hemoglobinopathies, especially S—C, S—S and C—C disease. The combination of hemoglobinopathies and pregnancy is hazardous for both mother and child. Secondary hemolysis may be observed after incompatable blood transfusions and in overwhelming septicemias.

Jaundice occurring in severe pyelonephritis during pregnancy (probably due to septicemia) has nearly disappeared since the advent of the antibiotics. A new syndrome has replaced it: jaundice in tetracycline toxicity used in the treatment of pyelonephritis during pregnancy. This toxic liver damage is often fatal. Postmortem examination reveals a diffuse fatty metamorphosis of the liver. So far it has not been seen in nonpregnant subjects.

Jaundice due to delayed chloroform poisoning and jaundice in criminal abortions are mainly of historic interest.

A second group of diseases, "jaundice *of* pregnancy", consists of disorders caused by pregnancy itself or occurring in typical complications linked to pregnancy.

Intrahepatic cholestasis of pregnancy is an entity benign to both mother and child, but has a marked tendency to recur in successive gestations. There are no prodromal symptoms such as in viral hepatitis or as in drug-induced intrahepatic cholestasis. The disease is characterized by often violent pruritus and mild jaundice, both disappearing usually within two weeks after spontaneous or induced delivery. Onset of jaundice is generally after the 22nd week of gestation but may occur as early as the 7th week. Biochemically there is an obstructive pattern with an increase of serum bilirubin, alkaline phosphatase, cholesterol, and alpha-2 and beta globulins on electrophoresis. Transaminases are mildly to moderately increased. Abnormal bromsulfalein retention is present, but galactose tolerance is normal. Flocculation and turbidity reactions are normal. Radiological gallbladder examinations show no filling during jaundice, but bile flow in the extrahepatic biliary system is unimpaired. Liver biopsy shows only a mild and usually focal or irregular cholestasis with no evidence of liver cell damage.

Acute fatty metamorphosis of pregnancy is a rare disorder with a very high mortality. Histologically it presents as a diffuse fatty change of the liver with the exception of a sharply defined rim of normal liver cells around the portal tract. There is no necrosis or inflammation. Clinically the disease resembles fulminant viral hepatitis. Onset of symptoms is always after the 30th and in the majority after the 36th week of gestation. Sudden and persistent vomiting is followed by abdominal pains, jaundice and tachycardia. There is no fever. The patient rapidly becomes somnolent and vomiting assumes a coffee-ground aspect. Premature labor sets in, the patient delivers a stillborn child, lapses into coma and dies with a terminal temperature elevation usually 1 to 7 days post partum. Few patients have survived. Two survivals occurred after early Caesarian section. Serum bilirubin rarely surpasses 10 mg per 100 ml, alkaline phosphatase and transaminases are moderately elevated, prothrombin time is markedly prolonged, white cell counts vary between 20,000 and 30,000, and flocculation and turbidity reactions are normal. Hypoglycemic episodes may occur and oliguria with azotemia is not uncommon. A few patients had associated pancreatitis.

Both intrahepatic cholestasis of pregnancy and acute fatty metamorphosis of pregnancy do not occur outside of gestation and in both the etiology is unknown.

Hyperemesis gravidarum is occasionally associated with mild jaundice and rarely with pruritus. Pathological bile components may be present in the urine, the transaminases may be slightly elevated and occasionally the flocculation tests are positive. Histological liver changes are absent or nonspecific. Jaundice in hyperemesis has no prognostic significance and clears with the cessation of vomiting.

Toxemia of pregnancy is associated with a high incidence of abnormal "liver function tests". Flocculation tests are positive in about half the cases. Alkaline phosphatase is elevated and parallels the clinical course. Transaminases are increased in the more severe cases. Jaundice is rare and carries a grave prognostic outlook. Histological liver changes are impressive at postmortem examination, but absent or minor in liver biopsies. These changes appear to be a terminal event, reflect the basic vascular disorder, and cannot be implicated in the genesis of the disturbed liver function tests.

The only disease in which an induced termination of pregnancy appears indicated because of jaundice, is acute fatty metamorphosis of pregnancy. In order to save the patient it should be performed very early after the onset of symptoms. An interruption of pregnancy may become necessary in toxemia but indications are based on general obstetric principles. Interruption of pregnancy may also be indicated in some cases of hemolysis not responding to medical treatment, but the decision is based on the degree of anemia and not on the presence of jaundice. Interruption is definitely not indicated in intrahepatic cholestasis of pregnancy, drug-induced cholestasis, familial hyperbilirubinemias, pyelonephritis and tetracycline toxicity. The course of viral hepatitis and liver cirrhosis is not altered by interruption of pregnancy and surgery is poorly tolerated in the severe cases in both diseases. Jaundice due to common duct stones is handled according to usual medical and surgical principles.

PART III contains a review on recurrent jaundice during pregnancy. A total of 132 cases are reported in the world literature. For the purpose of this review the cases have been divided into 6 categories according to their documentation (see Table 10). In 43 cases the diagnosis of intrahepatic cholestasis of pregnancy has been accepted (categories I and II). In 28 cases a different disease entity is responsible for recurrent jaundice (category VI). In 61 cases documentation is insufficient for a critical evaluation (categories III—V). In addition, 267 cases of non-recurrent intrahepatic cholestasis of pregnancy are briefly mentioned (category VII).

The terminology formerly used for recurrent intrahepatic cholestasis of pregnancy includes icterus gravidarum, jaundice of pregnancy, idiopathic jaundice of pregnancy, recurrent jaundice of pregnancy, benign jaundice of pregnancy, idiopathic hepatopathy of pregnancy, obstetric hepatosis, endogenous hepatotoxemia of pregnancy and cholestatic jaundice of pregnancy.

In 14 reports covering 23 patients the diagnosis of intrahepatic cholestasis of pregnancy is based on liver biopsies and

can be accepted beyond reasonable doubt (category I). Adequate laboratory examinations and details on clinical course are reported in 18 of these cases (category I A). These patients underwent a total of 70 gestations, in 47 of which the full syndrome with pruritus and jaundice occurred. The 47 pregnancies form the basis for establishing criteria of diagnosis in this disease.

Liver biopsies reveal only a mild centroacinar cholestasis, which is focal or irregular. Some bile canaliculi contain bile plugs. They are of normal caliber or slightly dilated. The surrounding liver cells contain biliary pigment. The liver cells are intact, as are the portal fields. There is no inflammation. Minor changes are consistent with those seen in uncomplicated pregnancies. Macroscopical findings in 10 patients undergoing surgical laparatomies were considered normal. Only one patient had gall bladder stones. In none was extrahepatic bile flow impaired. Radiological gallbladder examinations show no filling during jaundice and are normal after its subsidence.

Pruritus precedes jaundice usually by 1 to 2 weeks, in rare instances by up to 22 weeks. Itching is violent, involves the trunk and/or the extremities and leads to insomnia. Mean onset of jaundice is in the 26th week with an observed range between the 7th and the 39th week. Median duration of jaundice from its onset to spontaneous delivery is 6 weeks, and mean duration 8.1 weeks, with an observed range from 1 to 33 weeks. There are no prodromal symptoms such as in viral hepatitis. Apart from itching there are no general symptoms. General well-being is not impaired. Physical examination is normal except for the presence of jaundice and scratch marks. After delivery, whether spontaneous or induced, jaundice disappears within 1 to 2 weeks in the majority of patients, but may last in some up to 4 weeks postpartum. Itching subsides before jaundice. Recovery is complete after delivery.

Peak serum bilirubin is below 8.4 mg per 100 ml in all and below 6 mg per 100 ml in most cases. The direct-reacting bilirubin constitutes the major fraction. Urobilinogen is never absent from the urine. Urobilin and bilirubin are usually present. Bilirubinuria may be transient and can be missed. Alkaline phosphatase is increased to peak levels of 28 Bodansky units and serum cholesterol to maximally 590 mg per 100 ml. One or both these parameters may be normal in an occasional case. Serum electrophoresis shows an increase in alpha-2 and beta-globulins and a decrease in serum albumin. Gamma globulins are always lower than beta-globulins. Flocculation and turbidity test are normal. Prothrombin time may be prolonged when jaundice is of long duration. This is due to a deficiency in the Vitamin K dependent coagulation factors II, VII and X. Serum transaminases are elevated up to 250 units and reached 900 units in a single instance. Bromsulfalein retention at 45 minutes is between 10 and 25 %. Galactose tolerance is normal. There is no evidence of hemolysis.

After delivery there is a rapid decline of serum bilirubin and serum transaminases, while alkaline phosphatase may continue to rise for 4 to 10 days post partum. There are no obstetrical complications. In cases with prolonged prothrombin time blood loss during delivery may be excessive. The overall incidence of premature deliveries is high. Interestingly enough, premature delivery is confined to about one third of the patients while the others deliver at term. Premature delivery appears to be independent of jaundice per se. It may be caused by the same metabolic disturbance which also causes intrahepatic cholestasis. Child survival depends on the degree of maturity. No baby was icteric.

In successive pregnancies the syndrome may increase or decrease in severity or may present repeatedly with the same intensity. Clinical course regarding onset of jaundice and date of delivery is similar in many patients.

Treatment consists in the prophylactic application of Vitamin K and in the administration of cholestyramine to relieve itching. Neither diet nor bed rest are necessary and the patient may continue her usual daily life.

In some instances there are 2 or more cases of recurrent intrahepatic jaundice of pregnancy in close relatives. No antecedent liver disease is responsible for its occurrence.

Pruritus gravidarum appears to be a forme fruste of the full syndrome, and may show similar changes in alkaline phosphatase, serum cholesterol and serum transaminases.

The pathogenesis of intrahepatic cholestasis of pregnancy is unknown. Clinical cholestasis (itching) and functional cholestasis (alkaline phosphatase, cholesterol, electrophoresis) is marked, but structural cholestasis (liver biopsy) is minimal. "Physiological" derangement of liver function in normal pregnancy, pruritus gravidarum and intrahepatic cholestasis of pregnancy appear to be but increasing manifestations of the same basic disorder, and intrahepatic cholestasis of pregnancy is considered to be but an exaggeration of a "normal" process during gestation.

The differential diagnosis of recurrent jaundice during pregnancy is given in Table 23. Recurrent jaundice during pregnancy may probably occur in all benign disorders causing jaundice during pregnancy. Documented examples have been published for hemolytic jaundice, familial non-hemolytic jaundice, post-hepatitic hyperbilirubinemia, gall stone obstruction of the common bile duct, jaundice in severe pyelonephritis and jaundice in hyperemesis gravidarum. Cases with serum bilirubin levels above 10 mg per 100 ml represent mostly exacerbations of chronic anicteric hepatitis under the stress of pregnancy. Recurrent jaundice during pregnancy may be due to different diseases in successive gestations, for instance hepatitis in the first and hemolytic jaundice in the second gestation, or the etiology may be mixed in a single gestation, for instance hepatitis combined with hemolysis. Six recorded cases in the literature could not be classified at all.

The diagnosis of intrahepatic cholestasis of pregnancy should only be made when the criteria outlined above are met and when the differential diagnosis of recurrent jaundice during pregnancy has been carefully considered.

REFERENCES

*** cases of recurrent intrahepatic cholestasis of pregnancy with liver biopsy (category I).
** cases of recurrent intrahepatic cholestasis of pregnancy without liver biopsy but adequate laboratory data (category II).
* cases of recurrent jaundice during pregnancy with inadequate documentation (categories III— V).
° cases of non-recurrent intrahepatic cholestasis of pregnancy (category VII).
+ cases with recurrent jaundice during pregnancy of an etiology other than recurrent intrahepatic cholestasis of pregnancy (category VI).

ABRAMS, F. R. Cirrhosis of the liver in pregnancy. A review of the literature and report of a case with electrophoretic studies. Obstet. Gynec. 10, 451—456, 1956.

ADNO, J. Liver cirrhosis and pregnancy. Report of a case following spleno-renal shunt. South African M. J. 31, 1189—1191, 1957.

* AHLFELD, F. Icterus gravidarum. Berichte u. Arbeiten aus der Geb. Gyn. Klinik zu Giessen 1881—1882, pp. 148—153.

* AHLFELD, F. Lehrbuch der Geburtshilfe. W. Grunow. Leipzig 1898, 2. Aufl. p. 242.

AHRENS, E. H., PAYNE, M. H., KUNKEL, H. G., EISENMENGER, W. J. and BLANDHEIM, S. H. Primary biliary cirrhosis. Medicine 29, 299—364, 1950.

+ ALBANO, V. and ALBANO, S. B. L'epatite virale in gravidanza. Sicilia Sanit. 4, 95—116 1962.

ALEX, R. Ikterus in der Schwangerschaft (Ein kasuistischer Beitrag). Zbl. Gynäk. 73, 1324—1351, 1951.

ANTIA, F. P., BHARADWAJ, T. P., WATSA, M. C. and MASTER, J. Liver in normal pregnancy, pre-eclampsia and eclampsia. Lancet 2, 776—778, 1958.

ARFWEDSON, H. Graviditetsklåda. Svenska Läk. Tidningen 50, 1685—1689, 1953.

ARFWEDSON, H. General pruritus in pregnancy. Symptom of liver dysfunction. Obstet. Gynec. 7, 274—276, 1956.

ARFWEDSON, H. and v. STUDNITZ, W. Ueber bei Schwangerschaftspruritus auftretende Veränderungen des Lipoprotein-, Lipoid- und Proteingehaltes im Serum. Klin. Wschr. 34, 183—185, 1956.

ASHTON, D. L. Banti's disease complicating the puerperium. Am. J. Obstet. Gynec. 28, 280—281, 1934.

BAENS, A. and ESPINOLA, N. Acute yellow atrophy of the liver in pregnancy: report of cases. J. Philippine Med. Ass. 17, 679—685, 1937.

° BARRY, A. P. and O'DWYER, E. Hepatitis in pregnancy. Irish J. Med. Sci. 6, 419—424, 1955.

BEAN, W. B. The cutaneous arterial spider. A survey. Medicine 24, 243—331, 1945.

BEAN, W. B., COGSWELL, R., DEXTER, M. and EMBICK, J. F. Vascular changes of the skin in pregnancy. Vascular spiders and palmar erythema. Surg. Gynec. Obstet. 88, 739—752, 1949.

BEARN, A. G., KUNKEL, H. G. and SLATER, R. J. Problem of chronic liver disease in young women. Amer. J. Med. 21, 3—15, 1956.

BECK, E. and CLARK, L. C. Plasma alkaline phosphatase. II. Normal data for pregnancy. Amer. J. Obstet. Gynec. 60, 731—740, 1950.

* BECKING, A. G. T. Icterus gravidarum. Bijdrage tot de pathologie der zwangerschap. Tijdschr. voor Verlosk. en Gynaec. 7, 275—284, 1896.

*** BELVEDERI, C. and FINOTTI, A. Sulla patogenesi dell'ittero ricorrente gravidico. Riv. Ital. Ginec. 45, 108—123, 1961.

BENARON, H. B. W., DORR, E. M., RODDICK, W. J., JOHNSON, R. P., GOSSACK, L. and TUCKER, B. E. The use of chlorpromazine in the obstetric patient: a preliminary report. I. In the treatment of nausea and vomiting of pregnancy. Amer. J. Obstet. Gynec. 69, 776—779, 1955.

+ BENEDICT, H. Zur Kenntnis des Schwangerschaftsikterus. Dtsch. med. Wschr. 28, 296—297, 1902.

BENNET, A. G., KUNIN, A. S. and WALLACE, H. J. Liver disease in pregnancy: report of a case complicated by jaundice and cirrhosis with a review of the literature. Obstet. Gynec. Survey 18, 919—934, 1963.

*** BÉRAUD, C., BROUQUET, MARTIN, C., PACCALIN and TRAISSAC, F. J. L'ictère récidivant de la grossesse. Arch. Mal. Appar. Dig. 52, 256—261, 1963.

BJERREGAARD, P. C. Tilfaelde of Svangerskabs-Ikterus. Ugeskrift for Läger. 5. R. XI, 895—898, 1904.

BODANSKY, M., CAMPBELL, K. and BALL, E. Changes in serum calcium, inorganic phosphorus and phosphatase activity in the pregnant woman. Amer. J. Clin. Path. 9, 36—51, 1939.

+ BOQUIEN, Y., GUILLON, J., LERAT, M. and LENNE, C. Les ictères de la grossesse. Gynéc. Obstét. (Paris) 60, 562—584, 1961.

* BOREEL, M. Over een geval van icterus gravidarum. Ned. Tijdschr. Geneesk. 68, 1018—1022, 1924.

BORGLIN, N. E. Serum transaminase activity in uncomplicated and complicated pregnancy and in newborns. J. Clin. Endocrin. 18, 872—877, 1958.

+ BRAUER, L. Ueber Graviditäts-Haemoglobinurie. Münch. med. Wschr. 49, 825—826, 1902.

* BRAUER, L. Ueber Graviditätsikterus. Zbl. Gynäk. 27, 787—789, 1903.

BRET, J. and SÉNÈZE, J. Les ictères au cours de la grossesse. Rev. int. Hépat. 7, 557—578, 1957.

BRET, J. and SÉNÈZE, J. Les ictères au cours de la grossesse. Rev. pract. (Paris) 8, 963—973, 1958.

BROCQ, PORTES and VARANGOT, Ictère chronique par retention d'origine lithiasique au cours de la grossesse; cure chirurgicale; guérison. Gynéc. Obstét. (Paris) 42, 120—121, 1942.

+ BROMBERG, Y. M., TOAFF, R. and EHRENFELD, E. Acute crises in chronic hemolytic anemia induced by pregnancy. J. Obstet. Gynaec. Brit. Emp. 55, 325—329, 1948.

° BROWN, D. F., PORTA, E. A. and REDER, J. Idiopathic jaundice of pregnancy. Clinical, chemical and ultrastructural hepatic changes in three cases. Arch. Int. Med. 111, 592—606 1963.

BRUNO, M. S. and OBER, W. B. Jaundice at the end of pregnancy. Clinico-pathological conference. New York State J. Med. 62, 3792—3800, 1962.

BUDD, G. bearbeitet von Henoch, E. H. Die Krankheiten der Leber. A. Hirschwald, Berlin, 1846, p. 432.

BURSLEM, R. W., GARDIKAS, C. and ISRAELS, M. C. G. Liver cirrhosis and pregnancy. J. Obstet. Gynaec. Brit. Emp. 59, 777—782, 1952.

*** CAHILL, K. M. Hepatitis in pregnancy.
* Surg. Gynec. Obstet. 114, 545—552, 1962.

CANTAROW, A., STUCKERT, H. and GARTMAN E. Studies of hepatic function. IV. Hepatic function during pregnancy. Amer. J. Obstet. Gynec. 29, 36—43, 1935.

CAROLI, J., PARAF, A. and ZERVOYANNIS, S. Forme cholostatique pure des hépatites ictérogènes. Rev. med. Suisse rom. 73, 929—963, 1953.

* CAROLI, J., PUYO, G. and RAMPON, Re-
+ marques sur les hépatites ictérigènes de la grossesse. Semaine Hôp. Paris 30, 1692—1699, 1954.

CATTAN, R. and CATTAN, A. Ictère et grossesse. Rev. int. Hépat. 9, 399—416, 1959.

CAYLA, J. and FABRE, F. La phosphatase sérique pendant la gestation. Compte rend. Soc. Biol. 120, 748—750, 1935.

+ CHABROL, E. Les ictères. Masson & Cie. Paris 1932, p. 266.

CHRISTHILF, S. M. and BONSNES, R. W. Liver function during pregnancy and the puerperium, as measured by the cephalin-cholesterol flocculation, the thymol turbidity and the bromsulfalein tests. Amer. J. Obstet. Gynec. *59*, 1100—1104, 1950.

Clinicopathologic conference. Fulminating liver disease in a pregnant woman at term. Amer. J. Med. *35*, 231—240, 1963.

COMBES, B., SHIBATA, H., ADAMS, R., MITCHELL, B. D. and TRAMMELL, V. Alterations in sulfobromophthalein sodium removal mechanisms from blood during normal pregnancy. J. Clin. Invest. *42*, 1431—1442, 1963.

° COMERFORD, J. B. The diagnosis and treatment of hepatitis in pregnancy. J. Obstet. Gynaec. Brit. Cwlth. *69*, 1022—1028, 1962.

CORCOS, A. Ictère grave et grossesse (A propos de 8 cas). Presse méd. *62*, 544—(544) 1954.

CORYELL, M. N., BEACH, E. F., ROBINSON, A, R., MACY, I. G. and MACK, H. C. Metabolism of women during the reproductive cycle. XVII. Changes in electrophoretic patterns of plasma proteins throughout the cycle and following delivery. J. Clin. Invest. *29*, 1559—1567, 1950.

CREMONA, G. F. and VOGHERA, G. Considerazioni cliniche sulle epatopatie itterigene in gravidanza. Minerva Ginec. *14*, 1199 —1212, 1962.

CRISMER, R. Ictère hémolytique acquis toxigravidique. Acta gastro-enterol. Belg. *15*, 549—553, 1952.

CRISP, W. E., MIESFELD, R. L. and FRAJOLA, W. J. Serum glutamic oxalacetic transaminase levels in the toxemias of pregnancy. Obstet. Gynec. *13*, 487—497, 1959.

CROSS, R. C. A study of various liver function tests in normal pregnancy. Amer. J. Obstet. Gynec. *18*, 800—807, 1929.

CULLINAN, E. R. Idiopathic jaundice (often recurrent) associated with subacute necrosis of the liver. St. Bart. Hosp. Rep. *69*, 55—142, 1936.

CURTIS, E. M. Pregnancy in sickle-cell anemia, sickle-cell hemoglobin C disease, and variants thereof. Amer. J. Obstet. Gynec. *77*, 1312—1323, 1959.

DAMESHEK, W. and SCHWARTZ, S. O. Acute hemolytic anemia (acquired hemolytic icterus, acute type). Medicine *19*, 231—327, 1940.

DAY, E. M. A. and HELLESTRAND, A. L. An investigation of liver function in normal pregnancy and in the late toxemias of pregnancy. Australian Med. J. *2*, 326—329, 1947.

DECAUDIN, E. Concommitance des maladies du foie et des reins et en particulier des reins dans l'ictère. V. A. Delahaye et Cie. Paris. 1878, pp. 117.

DE GROOTE, J., GOUBEAU, P. and VANDENBROUCKE, J. Ictère cholostatique récidivant. Acta gastroenterol. Belg. *23*, 747—755, 1960.

DENNING, H. and BRUCKMANN, R. Virushepatitis und Schwangerschaft. Münch. med. Wschr. *103*, 1817—1821, 1961.

DIECKMANN, W. J. The toxemias of pregnancy. C. V. Mosby Company, St. Louis, 2nd ed. 1952.

DIECKMANN, W. J., SMITTER, R. C. and POTTINGER, R. E. Liver function studies in normal and toxemic pregnancy. Surg. Gynec. Obstet. *92*, 598—600, 1951.

DIECKMANN, W. J. and POTTINGER, R. E. Serial studies of the cephalin flocculation and thymol turbidity tests in pregnant patients. Amer. J. Obstet. Gynec. *68*, 1581—1583, 1954.

DIETEL, H. Die Leberfunktionsprüfung in der Schwangerschaft. Ztschr. Geburtsh. Gynäk. *113*, 209—254, 1936.

DIETEL, H. Das Bild der Leber in der Schwangerschaft (dargestellt auf Grund bioptischer Untersuchungen). Ztschr. Geburtsh. Gynäk. *128*, 127—162, 1947.

DIETEL, H. Hepatitis epidemica und Schwangerschaft. Geburtsh. Frauenheilk. *12*, 525—534, 1952.

DIETEL, H. Störungen und Erkrankungen der weiblichen Geschlechtsorgane in ihren Beziehungen zur Leber und Gallenblase. in: Seitz. L. and Amreich, A.I. Biologie und Pathologie des Weibes. Ein Handbuch der Frauenheilkunde und Geburtshilfe. 2. Aufl. Bd. 6 Teil 3. Verlag Urban & Schwarzenberg, Berlin-München-Wien 1954.

*** DIETEL, H. Der idiopathische Schwanger-
  + schaftsikterus. Geburtsh. Frauenheilk. *22*, 505—510, 1962.

DILL, L. V. Acute yellow atrophy of the liver associated with pregnancy; a review of the literature and six cases. Obstet. Gynec. Surv. *5*, 139—158, 1950.

*** DÖLLE, W. and MARTINI, G. A. Gelbsucht mit Verschlussyndrom als Leitsymptom bei Virushepatitis, Arzneimittelschäden, in der Schwangerschaft und bei Neugeborenen. Acta hepato-splen. *6*, 138—155, 255—247, 1959.

DÖLLE, W. and MARTINI, G. A. Zusammenstellung von Arzneimitteln, die Leberschädigung mit und ohne Gelbsucht verursachen können. (Ergänzung) Acta hepato-splen. *9*, 74—85, 1962.

DOMINICI, G. Le malattie del fegato e delle vie biliari. F. Vallardi, Milano, 3. ed. Vol. 1 1960, p. 720—721.

DÖRFLER, R. Zur Frage der kindlichen Missbildungen infolge Erkrankung der Mutter an Hepatitis epidemica während der Schwangerschaft. Münch. med. Wschr. *99*, 1664—1667, 1957.

DÖRFLER, R. Ueber die Häufigkeit hepatischer Embryopathien. Aerztl. Wschr. *13*, 779—781 1958.

* DOWIE, R. A case of jaundice recurring in pregnancy. J. Obstet. Gynaec. Brit. Emp. *61*, 399—(399) 1954.

DUBIN, I. N. Chronic idiopathic jaundice. A review of fifty cases. Amer. J. Med. *24*, 268—292, 1958.

DUBIN, I. N., SULLIVAN, B. H., LE GOLVAN, P. C. and MURPHY, L. C. The cholostatic form of viral hepatitis. Experiences with viral hepatitis at Brooke Army Hospital during the years 1951 to 1953. Amer. J. Med. *29*, 55—72, 1960.

DUNCAN, C. and MACLACHLAN, G. R. Report of a case of yellow atrophy of the liver in the latter part of pregnancy, with recovery. Amer. J. Obstet. Gynec. *25*, 157—158, 1933.

DURST, M. and STRAUSS, B. Transaminasenbestimmungen in der Geburtshilfe. Geburtsh. Frauenheilk. *23*, 927—934, 1963.

DYSON, B. C. Fatty metamorphosis of the liver in pregnancy; report of a fatal case without jaundice. Bull. Ayer Clin. Lab. Penn. Hosp. *4*, 17—30, 1959.

EDWARDS, A. G. A case of obstetrical acute yellow atrophy of the liver. J. Obstet. Gynaec. Brit. Emp. *67*, 460—462, 1960.

ELLEGAST, H., GUMPESBERGER, G. and WEWALKA, F. Hepatitis in der Gravidität und Frühgeburt. Wien. klin. Wschr. *66*, 30—32, 1954a.

ELLEGAST, H., GUMPESBERGER, G., RISSEL, E. and WEWALKA, F. Virushepatitis und Gravidität. Häufigkeit und Schwere der Hepatitis. Wien. klin. Wschr. *66*, 42—48, 1954b.

ELLEGAST, H., GUMPESBERGER, G. and WEWALKA, F. Einfluss einer Hepatitis in der Schwangerschaft auf das Kind. Wien. klin. Wschr. *66*, 507—511, 1954 c.

ENRILE, R. R., ARELLANO, S. O., TAMAYO, J. G. and SANTOS, D. C. Jaundice in pregnancy. J. Philippine Med. Ass. *33*, 587—602, 1957.

* EPPINGER, H. Icterus gravidarum. in: Kraus, P. and Brugsch, T. Spezielle Pathologie und Therapie innerer Krankheiten, Bd. 6, 2. Hälfte, III. Teil, Urban & Schwarzenberg, Berlin/Wien, 1923, pp. 305—306.

EPPINGER, H. Die Leberkrankheiten. Allgemeine und spezielle Pathologie und Therapie der Leber. Julius Springer, Wien, 1937, pp. 532—535.

ERNAELSTEEN, D. and WILLIAMS, R. Jaundice due to Nitrofurantoin. Gastroenterology *41*, 590—593, 1961.

EUFINGER, H. and BADER, C. W. Pigmentstoffwechsel der Leber in der Schwangerschaft. Arch. Gynäk. *128*, 293—308, 1926.

EUFINGER, H. and BADER, C. W. Die Bedeutung der H.v.d.Berg'schen Probe in der Schwangerschaft, insbesondere bei Toxikosen. Zbl. Gynäk. *50*, 514—517, 1926.

+ EZÈS, H. and BOURDON, R. Les hépatites ictérigènes graves d'allure virale au cours de la gestation (Synthèse critique de 36 observations recueillies de 1952—1956). Gynéc. Obstét. (Paris) *55*, 288—311, 1956.

FERRU, M. L'ictère dans les vomissements graves de la grossesse. Thèse, Paris 1926.

FOUCHÉ, H. H. and SWITZER, P. K. Pregnancy with sickle cell anemia. Review of the literature and report of cases. Amer. J. Obstet Gynec. *58*, 468—477, 1949.

FOULK, W. T., BUTT, H. R., OWEN, C. A., WHITCOMB, F. F. and MASON, H. L. Constitutional hepatic dysfunction (Gilbert's Disease): its natural history and related syndromes. Medicine *38*, 25—46, 1959.

FRERICHS, F.T. Klinik der Leberkrankheiten. Verlag F. Vieweg, Braunschweig, 1858, Bd. I, pp. 200—201.

FRIEDBERG, V. Ueber die latenten Schwangerschaftshepatosen. Z. Geburtsh. Gynäk. *134*, 27—39, 1951.

FRIEDBERG, V. Die Leberfunktion in der Schwangerschaft. Acta hepato-splen. *7*, 214—229, 1960.

* FRIEDBERG, V. Ueber die Bedeutung der Leberfunktionsprüfungen in der Schwangerschaft. Geburtsh. Frauenheilk. *22*, 109—122, 1962.

FRIEDBERG, V. Die Leberfunktion in der Schwangerschaft. Münch. med. Wschr. *105*, 58—64, 1963.

FRIEDMAN, M. M., LAPAN, B. and TAYLOR, T. H. Variations of enzyme activities during normal pregnancy. Amer. J. Obstet. Gynec. *82*, 132—137, 1961.

FRUCHT, H. L. and METCALFE, J. Mortality and late results of infectious hepatitis in pregnant women. New Engl. J. Med. *25*, 1094—1096, 1954.

+ FRUHINSHOLZ, A. Á propos de la pyélite gravidique, un cas de syndrome pyélohépato-rénal récidivant à deux gestations successives. Bull. Soc. Obstét. Gynéc. *18*, 141—145, 1929.

* GABRIEL, H. and BERNARDIN, D. Treize observations d'ictère au cours de la grossesse. Bull. Féd. Gynéc. Obstét. Franç. *14*, 395—398, 1962.

GALL, E. A. and BRAUNSTEIN, H. Hepatitis with manifestations simulating bile duct obstruction (so-called "cholangiolitic hepatitis"). Amer. J. Clin. Path. *25*, 1113—1127, 1955.

GEBHARDT, W. F., VAN OMMEN, R. A., McCORMACK, L. J. and BROWN, C. H. Chlorpromazine jaundice. Clinical course, hepatic function tests, and pathological findings — summary of twenty cases. Arch. Int. Med. *101*, 1085—1093, 1958.

GERL, D. and BONOW, A. Zur Klinik und Differentialdiagnose des Ikterus der Schwangeren. Med. Klin. *59*, 1—6, 1954.

GOLDSTEIN, K. and CONTINO, C. A. Intrahepatic cholestasis of pregnancy. Bull. Millard Fillmore Hosp. *9*, 75—78, 1962.

*** GROS, H. Der recidivierende idiopathische Schwangerschaftsikterus. Dtsch. med. Wschr. *83*, 383—386, 1958.

GROS, H. Personal communication, 1964.

GUTTMACHER, A. F. Hyperemesis. in: Guttmacher, A.F. and Rovinsky J. J., pp. 166-169.

GUTTMACHER, A. F. and ROVINSKY, J. J. Medical, surgical and gynecological complications of pregnancy. Williams & Wilkins Company, Baltimore 1960.

*** HAEMMERLI, U. P. and WYSS, H. I. Re-
** current intrahepatic cholestasis of pregnancy Report of six cases, with liver biopsies in four. (Manuscript submitted for publication).

° HAEMMERLI, U. P. and WYSS, H. I. unpublished observations.

VON HARNACK, G. A. and MARTINI, G. A. Hepatitis und Schwangerschaft. Die Auswirkung der Hepatitis auf die Frucht. Dtsch. med. Wschr. *77*, 40—42, 1952.

HARTMANN, F. and SCHOEN, R. Hepatitis in der Schwangerschaft. Geburtsh. Frauenheilk. *15*, 305—312, 1955.

*** HAUSHEER, H. J. and LAUER, D. J. Recurrent jaundice of pregnancy. Report of a case. New Engl. J. Med. *267*, 1300—1301, 1962.

HAVERBACK, B. J. and WIRTSCHAFTER, S. K. Familial nonhemolytic jaundice with normal liver histology and conjugated bilirubin. New Engl. J. Med. *262*, 113—117, 1960.

HEROLD, L. Die Leberfunktion in der physiologischen Schwangerschaft und bei der Hyperemesis gravidarum. Arch. Gynäk. *168*, 509—524, 1939.

HESSELTINE, H. C. Splenomegaly with hepatic cirrhosis (Banti's syndrome) as a complication of pregnancy, with the report of a case. Amer. J. Obstet. Gynec. *20*, 77—80 1930.

HILL, J. H. Serum lactic dehydrogenase in cancer patients. J. Nat. Cancer Institute *18*, 307—313, 1957.

HOCH, H., MARRACK, J. R., RUSE, R. H. and HOCH, R. The composition of the blood of women during pregnancy and after delivery. J. Obstet. Gynaec. Brit. Emp. *55*, 1—16, 1948.

HOFBAUER, J. Beiträge zur Aetiologie und zur Klinik der Graviditätstoxicosen (Cholämie, Eklampsie, Hyperemese). Z. Geburtsh. Gynäk. *61*, 200—274, 1907.

* HOFFMAN, cited in MEUNIER, J. Essay critique sur l'ictère des femmes enceintes à propos de l'épidemie de Paris 1871—1872. Thèse, Paris 1872, p. 17

* HOLMER, A. J. M. Lever en zwangerschap. Ned. Tijdschr. Verlosk. en Gynaec. *32*, 296—308, 1927.

HORN, G. Observations on the aetiology of cholelithiasis. Brit. Med. J. *2*, 732—737, 1956.

HOUEL, P., FABREGOULE, M., GARES, R. and BOURDON, R. Les formes malignes de l'hépatite virale au cours de la gestation. Sem. Hôp. Paris *34*, 1037—1043, 1958.

HOYNCK VAN PAPENDRECHT, H. P. C. M. Leverfunctiestoornissen in het laatste trimester van de zwangerschap. Ned. Tijdschr. Verlosk. en Gynec. *57*, 403—410, 1957.

HSIA, D. Y., TAYLOR, R. G. and GELLIS, S. S. A long-term follow-up study on infectious hepatitis during pregnancy. J. Pediat. *41*, 13—17, 1952.

*** IKONEN, E. Jaundice in late pregancy. Acta
  * obstet. gynec. Scand. *43*, Suppl. 5, 1—130,
  ° 1964.
  +

IMPARATO, E. Gli itteri in gravidanza. Rass. int. Clin. Therap. *38*, 557—558, 1958.

INGERSLEV, M. and TEILUM, G. Biopsy studies on the liver in pregnancy. I. Normal histological features of the liver as seen on aspiration biopsy. Acta obstet. gynec. Scand. *25*, 339—351, 1945.

INGERSLEV, M. and TEILUM, G. Biopsy studies on the liver in pregnancy. II. Liver biopsy on normal pregnant women. Acta obstet. gynec. Scand. *25*, 352—360, 1945.

INGERSLEV, M. and TEILUM, G. Biopsy studies on the liver in pregnancy. III. Liver biopsy in albuminuria of pregnancy, eclampsism and eclampsia. Acta obstet. gynec. Scand. *25*, 361—376, 1945.

INGERSLEV, M. and TEILUM, G. Jaundice during pregnancy. Acta obstet. gynec. Scand. *31*, 74—89, 1951.

JAVERT, C. T. and MORRISON, R. C. Jaundice. II. Its relationsship to pregnancy. Texas J. Med. *47*, 137—141, 1951.

JEFFRIES, G. H. and SLEISENGER, M. H. Acute intrahepatic cholestasis. Med. Clin. N. America *44*, 623—632, 1960.

** JODKOWSKI, H. and CHOJECKA, B. Nawracajaca żoltaczka w przebiegu ciaży. Pol. Tyk. Lek. *16*, 891—893, 1961.

JOHN, G. G. and KNUDTSON, K. P. Chronic idiopathic jaundice; two cases occurring in siblings, with histochemical studies. Amer. J. Med. *21*, 138—142, 1956.

+ JUSTIN-BESANÇON, L., PEQUINOT, H., ETIENNE J. P. and PHILBERT, M. L'ictère gravidique récidivant. Rev. méd. Franç. *40*, 75—83, 1959.

KAHIL, M. E., FRED, H. L., BROWN, H. and DAVIS, J. S. Acute fatty liver of pregnancy. Report of two cases. Arch. Int. Med. *113*, 63—69, 1964.

KALK, H. Ueber die posthepatitische Hyperbilirubinämie. Gastroenterologia *84*, 207—225, 1955.

KASDON, S. C. Abdominal pruritus in pregnancy. Amer. J. Obstet. Gynec. *65*, 320—324, 1953.

** KATZ, R., VELASCO, M., MANZUR, F. and
° DONOSO, S. Ictericia del embarazo. Rev. Med. Chile *89*, 110—115, 1961.

KAUFMANN, C. Ueber die Schwangerschaftsleber. Z. Geburtsh. Gynäk. *99*, 582—588, 1931.

KAUFMANN, C. Ueber die Schwangerschaftsumstellung der Leberfunktion. Klin. Wschr. *11*, 493—495, 1932.

* KEHRER, E. Zur Lehre von der embryogenen Toxaemia gravidarum. Klin. Vorträge N.F. Nr 398, Serie *15*, 365—404, 1905.

KEHRER, E. Die Bedeutung des Ikterus in der Schwangerschaft für Mutter und Kind. Klinische und experimentelle Untersuchungen. Arch. Gynaec. *81*, 129—159, 1907

KELLOG, C. S. and WESP, J. E. Infectious hepatitis during pregnancy and its effect upon the fetus. Amer. J. Obstet. Gynec. *62*, 1153—1156, 1951.

*** KING, M. J. and KERRINS, J. F. Recurrent idiopathic jaundice of pregnancy. New Eng. J. Med. *268*, 1180—1182, 1963.

KLAJMAN, A. and EFRATI, P. Prolonged jaundice with unidentified pigment in liver cells. Lancet *1*, 538—539, 1955.

KLIER, E. Ikterus im Rahmen der Schwangerschaftsfrühtoxicose. Wien. klin. Wschr. *68*, 64—66, 1956.

KNUTSON, R. G., CORNATZER, W. E., MOORE, J. H. and NELSON, W. W. Serum lactic dehydrogenase and glutamic oxalacetic transaminase activities in normal pregnancy. J. Lab. Clin. Med. *51*, 773—777, 1958.

KRAUL, L. Lebercirrhose und Schwangerschaft. Zbl. Gynäk. *51*, 663—669, 1927.

KUBLI, F. Transaminase, Milchsäuredehydrogenase und alkalische Phosphatase in der Spätschwangerschaft, unter der Geburt und bei Toxikose. Gynaecologia *151*, 72—74, 1961.

KÜHN, H. A. Ikterus durch intrahepatische Cholestase bei Brüdern. Acta hepato-splen. *9*, 229—245, 1962.

KUVIN, S. F. and BRECHER, G. Differential neutrophil counts in pregnancy. New Engl. J. Med. *266*, 877—878, 1962.

LABBY, D. H. Liver function and primary liver disease in pregnancy. Gen. Pract. *22*, 114—123, 1960.

LABO, G., FACCI, M. and RAITI, F. Le epatiti acute itterigene in gravidanza. Studio funzionale del fegato gravidico. Bologna Med. *5*, 745—768, 1959.

+ LACOMME, M. Ictère et gestation. Maternité *6*, 47—58, 1957.

+ LANTUÉJOUL, P. and CHAMBRAUD, R. Accouchements prématurés à répétition par insuffisance hépatique. Gynéc. Obstét. (Paris) *53*, 305—308, 1954.

LARGE, A. M., LOFSTROM, J. E. and STEVENSON, C. S. Gallstones and pregnancy. Arch. Surg. *78*, 966—968, 1959.

LASCANO, J. C. and PEREYRA, J. C. Gran ascitis por cirrosis hepática y embarazo. Prensa méd. Argent. *23*, 1794—1800, 1936.

° LAURIJSSENS, M. and DEMEULENAERE, L. Idiopathische icterus bij de zwangerschap. Belg. Tijdschr. Geneesk. *18*, 946—952, 1962.

+ LEBON, J., CLAUDE, R., TRICOIRE, J., GALLEY P. and LEUTENEGGER, M. Ictère gravidique récidivant. Algérie Méd. *65*, 235—244, 1961.

LEPAGE, F. Contribution à l'étude de la pyélonéphrite dite «gravido-toxique». Thèse, Paris 1934.

LEWIS, P. L., TAKEDA, M. and WARREN, W. J. Obstetric acute yellow atrophy. Report of a case. Obstet. Gynec. *22*, 121—127, 1963.

LEY, H. and LIEBL, R. Ueber Ausmass und Häufigkeit von diffusen Hepatopathien nach einem Ikterus während der Schwangerschaft. Aerzt. Forschung *8*, 451—457, 1954.

LICHTMAN, S. S. Diseases of the liver, gallbladder and bile ducts. Lea and Febiger, Philadelphia, 3rd ed. 1953, pp. 636—644.

LINTON, E. B. and MILLER, E. C. Serum lactic dehydrogenase in pregnancy. Amer. J. Obstet. Gynec. *78*, 11—12, 1959.

*** LJUNGGREN, G. Kliniska synpunkter på
° ikterus under graviditet. Nord. med. *55*, 373—374, 1956.

LOCK, F. R., BURT, R. L. and LIDE, T. N. Hepatic failure in pregnancy. Amer. J. Obstet. Gynec. *65*, 859—872, 1953.

LONG, J. S., BOYSEN, H. and PRIEST, F. O. Infectious hepatitis and pregnancy. Amer. J. Obstet. Gynec. *70*, 282—287, 1955.

LOVE, W. and PEEL, E. L. Chlorpromazine jaundice in pregnancy. J. Obstet. Gynaec. Brit. Cwlth. *68*, 628—633, 1961.

+ LOVRICH, J. Zwei Fälle von Ikterus während der Schwangerschaft. Zbl. Gynäk. *28*, 776—(776) 1904.

LOWENSTEIN, L., BRUNTON, L., YANG-SHU, H. and MILAD, A. A. Folic acid and Vitamin B$_{12}$ deficiency in megaloblastic anemia of pregnancy. Amer. J. Dig. Dis. (NS) *7*, 984—985, 1962.

MACK, H. C., SEGAR, L. F., ROBINSON, A. R., WISEMAN, M. E. and MOGER, E. Z. Eletrophoretic patterns of plasma proteins in pregnancy. II. Pregnancy complicated by liver disease. Obstet. Gynec. *1*, 204—211, 1953.

** McALLISTER, J. E. and WADDELL, J. M. Recurring idiopathic jaundice in pregnancy: case report. Amer. J. Obstet. Gynec. *84*, 62—64, 1962.

McNair, R. D. and Jaynes, R. V. Alterations in liver function during normal pregnancy. Amer. J. Obstet. Gynec. *80*, 500—505, 1960.

* Magnani, L. Sull'ittero recidivante della gravidanza. Riv. ital. Ginec. *9*, 801—816, 1929.

Mansell, R. V. Infectious hepatitis in the first trimester of pregnancy and its effect on the fetus. Amer. J. Obstet. Gynec. *69*, 1136—1139, 1955.

Martin, R. and Ferguson, F. C. Infectious hepatitis associated with pregnancy. A report of four cases. New Engl. J. Med. *237*, 114—117, 1947.

Martini, G. Hepatitis und Schwangerschaft. Schweiz. Z. Allg. Path. *16*, 475—482, 1953.

Martini, G. A., von Harnack, G. A. and Napp. J. H. Hepatitis und Schwangerschaft. Die Auswirkung der Hepatitis auf die Mutter. Dtsch. med. Wschr. *78*, 661—665, 1953.

Mason, D. G. Acute fatty metamorphosis of the liver associated with pregnancy (C.P.C.) Northwest. Med. *57*, 456—462, 1958.

Mason, J. M. and Wróblewski, F. Serum glutamic oxalacetic transaminase activity in experimental and disease states. A review. Arch. Int. Med. *99*, 245—252, 1957.

* Mayer, A. Schwangerschaftsikterus als echte eingeschlechtliche Krankheit. Med. Klinik *2*, 1169—1172, 1906.

Mazad, R., Moissinac, J. and Labegorre, J. L'hépatite ictérigène de la grossesse. Méd. trop. (Marseille) *19*, 7—22, 1959.

* Meeroff, M. Ictericias del embarazo. Prensa med. Argent. *48*, 3313—3320, 1961.

Meinhold. Ein weiterer Fall von Schwangerschaftshämoglobinurie. Münch. med. Wschr. *50*, 166—166, 1903.

Meranze, T., Meranze, D. R. and Rothman, M. M. Blood phosphatase in pregnancy. Amer. J. Obstet. Gynec. *33*, 444—450, 1937.

Merletti, C. Urobilinurie bei Schwangeren und Vermehrung derselben in Fällen endouterinen Fruchttodes. Zbl. Gynäk. *26*, 417—421, 1902.

Metzger, L. Zur Casuistik des menstruellen Ikterus. Z. klin. Med. *53*, 149—152, 1904.

Meulengracht, E. A review of chronic intermittent juvenile jaundice. Quart. J. Med. *16*, 83—98, 1947.

Meunier, J. Essai critique sur l'ictère des femmes enceintes à propos de l'épidémie de Paris 1871—1872, Thèse, Paris, 1862, p. 17.

* Meyer, J. Ikterus und Schwangerschaft. Geburtsh. Frauenheilk. *15*, 1013—1019, 1955.

Meyer, M. L. A. Ictère de la grossesse. Semaine méd. *27*, 32—32, 1907.

Mickal, A. Infectious hepatitis in pregnancy. Amer. J. Obstet. Gynec. *62*, 409—414, 1951.

Millar, D. The significance of jaundice in pregnancy. J. Obstet. Gynaec. Brit. Emp. *61*, 405—405, 1954.

Millen, R. M. Jaundice during pregnancy. Brit. J. Clin. Pract. *11*, 341—345, 1957.

Moore, H. C. Acute fatty liver of pregnancy. Irish J. Med. Sci. *6*, 451—458, 1955.

Moore, H. C. Acute fatty liver of pregnancy. J. Obstet. Gynaec. Brit. Emp. *63*, 189—198, 1956.

*** Moore, H. C. Recurrent jaundice of preg-
** nancy. A type of intrahepatic cholestasis.
° Lancet *2*, 57—59, 1963.

Moore, R. M. and Hughes, P. K. Cirrhosis of the liver in pregnancy. A review of the literature and report of three cases. Obstet. Gynec. *15*, 753—756, 1960.

moore, W. J. Infectious hepatitis and pregnancy. Obstet. Gynec. *16*, 693—698, 1960.

Moyer, J. H., Kinross-Wright, V. and Finney, R. M. Chlorpromazine as a therapeutic agent in clinical medicine. Arch. Int. Med. *95*, 202—218, 1955.

Mukherjee, C. Plasma alkaline phosphatase in toxaemia of pregnancy. J. Indian Med. Ass. *21*, 43—52, 1951.

° Müller, S. and Felsch, G. Hepatitis und Hepatose in der Schwangerschaft. Med. Mschr. *17*, 300—305, 1963.

* Müllerheim, H. Diskussion zu Schaeffer, O., Zbl. Gynäk. *26*, 1125—1125, 1902.

Munnell, E. W. and Taylor, H. C. Liver blood flow in pregnancy — hepatic vein catheterization. J. Clin. Invest. *29*, 952—956, 1947.

° Myhre, J. Idiopathic jaundice of pregnancy. Report of a case. Amer. J. Dig. Dis. (NS) *8*, 852—855, 1963.

Nabriski, S., Zeloof, D., Fleishman, P. and Lewitus, Z. Pregnancy in cirrhosis of the liver. J. Obstet. Gynaec. Brit. Emp. *65*, 462—464, 1958.

Nardone, A. A., Stroup, P. E. and Gill, R. J. Acute fatty metamorphosis of the liver in pregnancy. Report of a case complicating toxemia in pregnancy. Amer. J. Obstet. Gynec. *80*, 258—262, 1960.

* Nason, E. N. Recurring jaundice in mother and infant. Brit. med. J. *1*, 989—990, 1910.

Niesert, W. Die Eisenbindungskapazität in der Schwangerschaft. Arch. Gynäk. *191*, 291—296, 1958.

° Nixon, W. C. W., Egeli, E. S., Laqueur,
+ W. and Yahya, O. Icterus in pregnancy. A clinico-pathological study including liver-biopsy. J. Obstet. Gynaec. Brit. Emp. *54*, 642—552, 1947.

Nürnberger, L. Zur Kenntnis der Leberfunktion am Ende der normalen Schwangerschaft. Arch. Gynaek. *153*, 1—25, 1933.

Ober, W. O. and Lecomte, P. M. Acute fatty metamorphosis of the liver associated with pregnancy. A distinctive lesion. Amer. J. Med. *19*, 743—758, 1955.

O'Connell, W. T. Hepatitis complicating pregnancy. Amer. J. Obstet. Gynec. *63*, 449—451, 1952.

O'Leary, J. A. and Bepko, F. J. Portocaval shunt performed during pregnancy. Report of a case. Obstet. Gynec. *20*, 243—246, 1962.

* Orellana, J. M., Gonzalez Rodriguez,
° A. and Aguirre, E. Ictericia benigna del embarazo. (Colostasis intrahepática del embarazo). Rev. med. Chile *89*, 676—679, 1961.

* Orellana, J. M. and Osorio, R. Intrahe-
° patic cholestasis of pregnancy. IInd World Congr. Gastroent. Munich 1962, *III*, 234—238, 1963.

+ Paschkis, K. Zur Frage des Terrain hépatique. Wien. klin. Wschr. *36*, 581—581, 1923.

Paul, W. M. Infectious hepatitis in pregnancy. Report of a case. Obstet. Gynec. *6*, 107—110, 1955.

* Pavel, I., Ceausi, G. and Gartenberg, A. L'ictère récidivant au cours des grossesses successives. Rev. int. Hépat. *7*, 317—324, 1957.

Peck, O. C., Rey, D. F. and Snell, A. M. Familial jaundice with free and conjugated bilirubin in the serum and without liver pigmentation. Gastroenterology *39*, 625—627, 1960.

* Pel, cited in Vignes, H. p. 47.

Peretz, A., Paldi, E., Brandstaedter, S. and Barzilai, D. Infectious hepatitis in pregnancy. Obstet. Gynec. *14*, 435—441, 1959.

* Perreau, P. Ictère récidivant de la grossesse. Arch. mal. appar. digest. *42*, 1394—1397, 1953.

** Perreau, P. and Rouchy, R. Ictère
* cholostatique récidivant de la grossesse.
+ Gynéc. Obstét. (Paris) *60*, 161—179, 1961.

Perreau, P. L'ictère cholostatique récidivant de la grossesse. in: «Les ictères» Actualités hép.-gastroent. hôp. Dieu, Masson·et Cie. Paris 1962, pp. 224—239.

Peters, R. L., Edmondson, H. A. and Kunelis, C. T. Acute fatty metamorphosis of the liver in pregnancy. (Abstract) J. Amer. Med. Ass. *180*, 767—767, 1962.

Pfau, D. Die Differenzierung der Plasmaproteine in der Schwangerschaft durch Elektrophorese. Geburtsh. Frauenheilk. *11*, 420—424, 1951.

Phatak, L. V. and Patil, K. A study of infective hepatitis in pregnancy. Indian J. Med. Sci. *10*, 593—601, 1956.

*** Pieragnoli, E., D'Antuono, G. and Tura, S. Ittero recidivante gravidico. Giorn. Clin. Med. *41*, 516—523, 1960.

Pirinoli, M. Hepatitis a virus y embarazo. Semana med. *64*, 1304—1309, 1957.

Popper, H. and Schaffner, F. Pathology of jaundice resulting from intrahepatic cholestasis. J. Amer. Med. Ass. *169*, 1447—1453, 1959.

Popper, H., Rubin, E. and Schaffner, F. The problem of primary biliary cirrhosis. Editorial. Amer. J. Med. *33*, 807—810, 1962.

POTTER, M. G. Observations of the gallbladder and bile during pregnancy at term. J. Amer. Med Ass. *106*, 1070—1074, 1936.

PUDER, H. Die akute Leberinsuffizienz in der Geburtshilfe. Münch. med. Wschr. *51*, 1713—1715, 1955.

* PUYO, G. Contribution à l'étude de certains
° ictères de la grossesse. Thèse, Paris 1953.
+

QUINCKE, H. and HOPPE-SEYLER, G. Die Krankheiten der Leber. A. Hölder, Wien, 1899, p. 133.

QUIRNO, N., NÖLTING, D. and DI FONZO, N. O. Gestosis a forma hepatica. Prensa méd. Argent. *35*, 2334—2337, 1948.

READ, A. E., HARRISON, C. V. and SHERLOCK, S. Chronic chlorpromazine jaundice with particular reference to its relationship to primary biliary cirrhosis. Amer. J. Med. *31*, 249—258, 1961.

REICHARD, H., WIQVIST, N. and YLLNER, S. Serum ornithyl carbamyl transferase activity in normal pregnancy and in pregnancy complicated by pruritus. Acta obstet. gynec. Scand. *40*, 244—251, 1961.

RICHMAN, A. The liver. in: Guttmacher, A. F. and Rovinsky, J. J. pp. 187—201.

RIMBACH, E. Die funktionelle Leistungsinsuffizienz in der Gravidität mit besonderer Berücksichtigung des nephrotoxischen Schwangerschaftsikterus. Geburtsh. Frauenheilk. *22*, 1264—1266, 1962.

+ RIMBACH, E. and BEICKERT, A. Hämolytischer Ikterus in der Schwangerschaft. Münch. med. Wschr. *97*, 876—877, 1955.

RIMBACH, E. and BONOW, A. Aenderungen der Transaminaseaktivität während der Schwangerschaft und im Wochenbett. Dtsch. med. Wschr. *84*, 1822—1825, 1959.

RISSMANN, P., Langdauernder Steinverschluss des Choledochus und des Diverticulum Vateri — transduodenale Operation in der Gravidität. Zbl. Gynaek. *33*, 689—691, 1909.

+ RISSMANN, P. Gibt es eine den Frauen eigentümliche Form der Gelbsucht? Eine literarisch-klinische Studie. Z. Geburtsh. Gynäk. *65*, 325—335, 1910.

RISSMANN, P. Milz und Leber in ihren Beziehungen zu den Stoffwechselstörungen der Schwangerschaft. Zbl. Gynäk. *41*, 641—643, 1917.

ROBERTSON, H. E. and DOCHAT, G. R. Pregnancy and gallstones. A collective review. Internat. Abstr. Surg. *78*, 193—204, 1944.

* ROLLESTON, H. D. Remarks on a case of recurring jaundice in four successive pregnancies, with fatal jaundice in three successive infants. Brit. Med. J. *1*, 864—865, 1910.

ROTH, L. G. Infectious hepatitis in pregnancy. Amer. J. Med. Sci. *225*, 139—146, 1953.

SALMON, G. W. and RICHMAN, E. E. Liver function in the newborn infant. J. Pediat. *23*, 522—533, 1943.

SAMUELS, B. Jaundice in pregnancy. A 10-year review at Touro infirmary. Obstet. Gynec. *17*, 103—108, 1961.

SANDERS, M. Hematologic complications. in: Guttmacher, A. F. and Rovinsky, J. J. pp. 396—413.

SAURER, A. Hepatitis epidemica in Gravidität und Wochenbett. Besondere Bedeutung einiger Beobachtungen für die Frauenheilkunde und interne Medizin. Mschr. Geburtsh. Gynäk. *115*, 16—33, 1943.

SCAGLIONE, S. Cirrosi di Laennec in gravidanza. Rev. ital. Ginec. *1*, 489—496, 1923.

+ SCHAEFFER, O. Ein Beitrag zur Aetiologie des wiederkehrenden Ikterus graviditatis. Mschr. Geburtsh. Gynäk. *15*, 897—920, 1902.

SCHAFFNER, F. Iatrogenic jaundice. J. Amer. Med. Ass. *174*, 1690—1695, 1960.

SCHAPIRO, R. H. and ISSELBACHER, K. J. Benign recurrent intrahepatic cholestasis. New Engl. J. Med. *268*, 708—711, 1963.

SCHICKELE, G. Beiträge zur Physiologie und Pathologie der Schwangerschaft (Schwangerschaftsleber. Atypische Eklampsie). Arch. Gynäk. *92*, 374—465, 1910.

SCHICKELE, G. Neuere Untersuchungen über die sogenannte Schwangerschaftsleber (hépatotoxémie gravidique). Zbl. Gynäk. *36*, 1325—1325, 1912.

SCHIFF, L., BILLING, B. H. and OIKAMA. Y. Familial non-hemolytic jaundice with conjugated bilirubin in the serum. A case study. New Engl. J. Med. *260*, 1315—1318, 1959.

SCHMID, M., HEFTI, M. L., GATTIKER, R., KISTLER, H. J. and SENNING, Å. Postoperative intrahepatic cholestasis — a benign postoperative jaundice. New Engl. J. Med. *272*, 545-550, 1965

+ SCHNEIDER, W. and FRAHM, H. Beitrag zur hämolytischen Krise und zur perniciosaähnlichen Anämie in der Schwangerschaft bei familiärem hämolytischem Ikterus. Dtsch. med. Wschr. *85*, 2074—2076, 1960.

SCHUBERT, R. and PETERS, H. Ikterus und Gravidität unter besonderer Berücksichtigung der Virushepatitis. Medizinische *23*, 315—318, 1954.

SCHULTZ, J. C., ADAMSON, J. S., WORKMAN, W. W. and NORMAN, T. D. Fatal liver disease after intravenous administration of tetracycline in high dosage. New Engl. J. Med. *268*, 999—1004, 1963.

* SCHWALM, M. Recidivierender Schwangerschaftsikterus. Zbl. Gynäk. *56*, 2098—2105, 1932.

SEITZ, L. Schwangerschaftsikterus. in: Döderlein, A. Handbuch der Geburtshilfe. Verlag J. F. Bergmann, Wiesbaden 1916, Band II, p. 215—217.

SEITZ, L. Schwangerschaftshepatocholepathien. in: Stoeckel, W. Lehrbuch der Geburtshilfe, 10. Auflage, Gustav Fischer, Jena, 1948, p. 539—541.

SENATOR, H. Ueber menstruelle Gelbsucht. Berl. klin. Wschr. *9*, 615—618, 1872.

** SEYDL, G. Der Ikterus in der Schwangerschaft. Medizin heute *11*, 528—531, 1962.

SHEEHAN, H. L. The pathology of hyperemesis and vomiting of late pregnancy. J. Obstet. Gynaec. Brit. Emp. *46*, 685—699, 1939.

SHEEHAN, H. L. The pathology of acute yellow atrophy and delayed chloroform poisoning. J. Obstet. Gynaec. Brit. Emp. *47*, 49—62, 1940.

* SHEEHAN, H. L. Jaundice in pregnancy. Amer. J. Obstet. Gynec. *81*, 427—440, 1961.

SHERLOCK, S. Diseases of the liver and biliary system. Blackwell, Oxford, 3rd ed. 1963 pp. 305—307, 491—495.

SIEGAL, I. A. Liver function in pregnancy. Amer. J. Obstet. Gynec. *14*, 300—312, 1927.

SIEGLER, A. M. and KEYSER, H. Acute hepatitis in pregacy: a report of ten cases and review of the literature. Amer. J. Obstet. Gynec. *86*, 1068—1073, 1963.

** SIMMONS, S. C. Recurrent jaundice in pregnancy. Lancet *2*, 60—61, 1963.

SLATER, R. J. Investigation of an infant born of a mother suffering from cirrhosis of the liver. Pediatrics *13*, 308—316, 1954.

SLAUGHTER, C. R. and KRANTZ, K. E. Cirrhosis of the liver complicating pregnancy; a presentation of 2 cases and a review of the literature. Amer. J. Obstet. Gynec. *86*, 1060—1067, 1963.

SOFFER, L. J. Bilirubin excretion as a test for liver function during normal pregnancy. Bull. Johns Hopkins Hosp. *52*, 365—375, 1933.

SPEERT, H., GRAFF, S. and GRAFF, A. M. Serum phosphatase relations in mother and fetus. Amer. J. Obstet. Gynec. *59*, 148—154, 1950.

STACEY, C. H., AZIMA, H., HUESTIS, D. W., HOWLETT, J. G. and HOFFMAN, M. M. Jaundice occurring during the administration of chlorpromazine. Canad. Med. Assoc. J. *73*, 386—392, 1955.

STANDER, H. J. and CADDEN, J. F., Acute yellow atrophy of the liver in pregnancy. Amer. J. Obstet. Gynec. *28*, 61—69, 1934.

STOKES, J., WOLMAN, I. J., BLANCHARD, M. C. and FARQUHAR, J. D. Viral hepatitis in the newborn: clinical features, epidemiology and pathology (Abstract) Amer. J. Dis. Child. *82*, 213—213, 1951.

STONE, M. L., LENDING, M., SLOBODY, L. B. and MESTERN, J. Glutamic oxalacetic transaminase and lactic dehydrogenase in pregnancy. Amer. J. Obstet. Gynec. *80*, 104—107, 1960.

VON STUDNITZ, W. Studies on serum lipids and lipoproteins in pregnancy. Scand. J. Clin. Lab. Invest. *7*, 329—335, 1955.

SULLIVAN, C. F., TEW, W. P. and WATSON, E. M. The bilirubin excretion test of liver function in pregnancy. J. Obstet. Gynaec. Brit. Emp. *41*, 347—368, 1934.

SUMMERSKILL, W. H. J. and WALSHE, J. M.

Benign recurrent intrahepatic «obstructive» jaundice. Lancet *2*, 686—690, 1959.

** SVANBORG, A. A study of recurrent jaundice
° in pregnancy. Acta obstet. gynec. Scand. *33*, 434—444, 1954.

*** SVANBORG, A. and OHLSSON, S. Recurrent
* jaundice of pregnancy. A clinical study of
° twenty-two cases. Amer. J. Med. *27*, 40—49, 1959.

SYNODINOS, E. Ictère et grossesse. Rev. Franç. Gynéc. Obstét. *58*, 313—344, 1963.

SYNODINOS, E. Ictère et grossesse. Gynéc. Obstét. (Paris) *62*, 107—134, 1963.

SYNODINOS, E., FRANGIADAKIS, L., PAPADOYIANAKIS, N. and STAVROPOULOS, A. Ictère et grossesse. Rev. Mèd. moyen Orient *19*, 84—92, 1962.

TAMAKI, H. T. and CARFAGNO, S. C. Chronic idiopathic jaundice with unidentified pigment in liver cells. Arch. Int. Med. *99*, 294—296, 1957.

TAYLOR, H. C. Infectious hepatitis in pregnancy. Connecticut Med. J. *16*, 587—591, 1952.

TENNEY, B. and KING, R. B. Pregnancy coincident with cirrhosis of the liver; report of a case. New Engl. J. Med. *208*, 1157—1160, 1933.

** THORLING, L. Jaundice in pregnancy. A
° clinical study. Acta med. Scand. Suppl.
+ *302*, 1—123, 1955.

TOPP, J. R. and CHARLES, B. Pruritus of pregnancy. A symptom of hepatic dysfunction, with a report of two cases. Canad. Med. Assoc. J. *85*, 724—726, 1962.

TYGSTRUP, N. Intermittent possibly familial intrahepatic cholestatic jaundice. Lancet *1*, 1171—1172, 1960.

+ TYLECOTE, F. E. Jaundice of pregnancy associated with jaundice in the offspring. Med. Chronicle *58*, 465—468, 1914.

TYSOE, F. W. and LOWENSTEIN, L. Blood volume and hematologic studies in pregnancy and the puerperium. Amer. J. Obstet. Gynec. *60*, 1187—1205, 1950.

° VAN WOERT, M. H. and KIRSNER, J. B. Idiopathic jaundice of pregnancy. Gastroenterology *40*, 633—635, 1961.

VARANGOT, J. Les ictères de la grossesse. in: «Les ictères», Actualités hép.-gastroent. Hôp. Dieu. Masson et Cie. Paris 1962, pp. 215—223.

VERHAGE, J. C. Hyperemesis gravidarum. Nederl. Tijdschr. Verlosk. Gynec. *43*, 36—74 1940.

* VERHAGE, J. C. Icterus in de zwangerschap. Nederl. Tijdschr. Verlosk. Gynec. *43*, 135—159, 1940.

VERMEHREN, E. Plasmaphosphatase während der Gravidität und der Laktation. Acta med. Scand. *100*, 254—266, 1939.

+ VIGNES, H. Maladies des femmes enceintes. II. Affections du foie, du pancréas. Maladies de la nutrition. Parois abdominale. Péritoine. Masson et Cie. Paris, 1935, p.42.

VINAY, Ch. Traité des maladies de la grossesse et des suites de couches. 1894, cited in Becking, A.G.T.

VINCENT, C. R. Jaundice in pregnancy. A review from the Charity Hospital, New Orleans, 1941—1956. Obstet. Gynec. *9*, 595—598, 1957.

* VON DEN VELDEN, R. Icterus gravidarum. Beitr. Geburtsh. Gynaek. *8*, 448—464, 1904.

WATSON, C. J. and HOFFBAUER, F. W. The problem of prolonged hepatitis with particular reference to the cholangiolitic type and to the development of cholangiolitic cirrhosis of the liver. Ann. Int. Med. *25*, 195—227, 1946.

WERNER, S. C., HANGER, F. M. and KRITZLER, R. A. Jaundice during methyl testosterone therapy. Amer. J. Med. *8*, 325—331, 1950.

WERTHER, J. L. and KORELITZ, B. Chlorpromazine jaundice. Analysis of twenty-two cases. Amer. J. Med. *22*, 351—366, 1957.

WEST, M. and ZIMMERMAN, H. J. Lactic dehydrogenase and glutamic oxaloacetic transaminase in normal pregnant women and newborn children. Amer. J. Med. Sci. *235*, 443—447, 1958.

WETSTONE, H. J., LA MOTTA, R. V., MIDDLEBROOK, L., TENNANT, R. and WHITE, B. V. Studies of cholinesterase activity. IV. Liver function in pregnancy: Values of certain standard liver function tests in normal pregnancy. Amer. J. Obstet. Gynec. *76*, 480—490, 1958.

* WEWALKA, F. Beitrag zur Hepatitis in der Schwangerschaft. Verhandl. Deutsch. Ges. Inn. Med. (63. Kongress 1957) *63*, 392—396, 1957.

WHALLEY, P. J., ADAMS, R. H. and COMBES, B. Tetracycline toxicity in pregnancy. Liver and pancreatic dysfunction. J. Amer. Med. Ass. *189*, 357—362, 1964.

WHITACRE, F. E. and FANG, L. Y. Fatty degeneration of the liver in pregnancy. Report of a case with recovery: chemical and histologic studies. J. Amer. Med. Ass. *118*, 1358—1364, 1942.

* WILKEN, H. Zur Frage der Leberschädigung in der Schwangerschaft. Dtsch. Gesundheitswes. *13*, 1432—1435, 1958.

WILKEN, H. Die »Leberclearance« mit Bromsulphalein in der Schwangerschaft und unter der Geburt. Zbl. Gynäk. *82*, 1804—1809, 1960.

WILLIAMS, H. M. Liver disease in pregnancy. Connecticut Med. J. *21*, 497—501, 1957.

WILLIAMS, R., CARTTER, M. A., SHERLOCK, S., SCHEUER, P. J. and HILL, K. R. Idiopathic recurrent cholestasis: a study of the function and pathological lesions in four cases. Quart. J. Med. (N.S.) *33*, 387—399, 1964.

VON WINCKEL, F. Icterus gravidarum. Lehrbuch der Geburtshilfe. von Keit & Co., Leipzig, 1893, 2. Aufl. pp. 239—241.

WINTER, J. T. Jaundice during pregnancy. Amer. J. Obstet. Gynec. *23*, 31—37, 1890.

YOUNG, J., KING, E. J., WOOD, E. and WOOTTON, I. D. P. A nutritional survey among pregnant women. J. Obstet. Gynaec. Brit. Emp. *53*, 251—259, 1946.

+ ZACHARIAE, F. A case of haemolytic anaemia induced by pregnancy. Acta obstet. gynec. Scand. *32*, 250—263, 1953.

ZONDEK, B. and BROMBERG, Y. M. Infectious hepatitis in pregnancy. J. Mt. Sinai Hosp. *14*, 222—243, 1947.